16

Elly Pear's

Fast Days & Feast Days

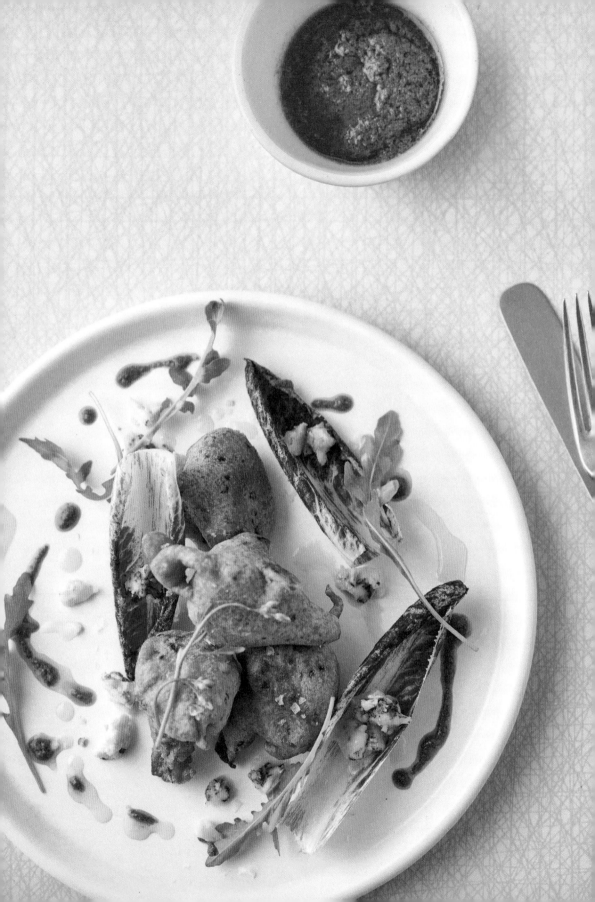

Elly Pear's

Fast Days & Feast Days

Contents

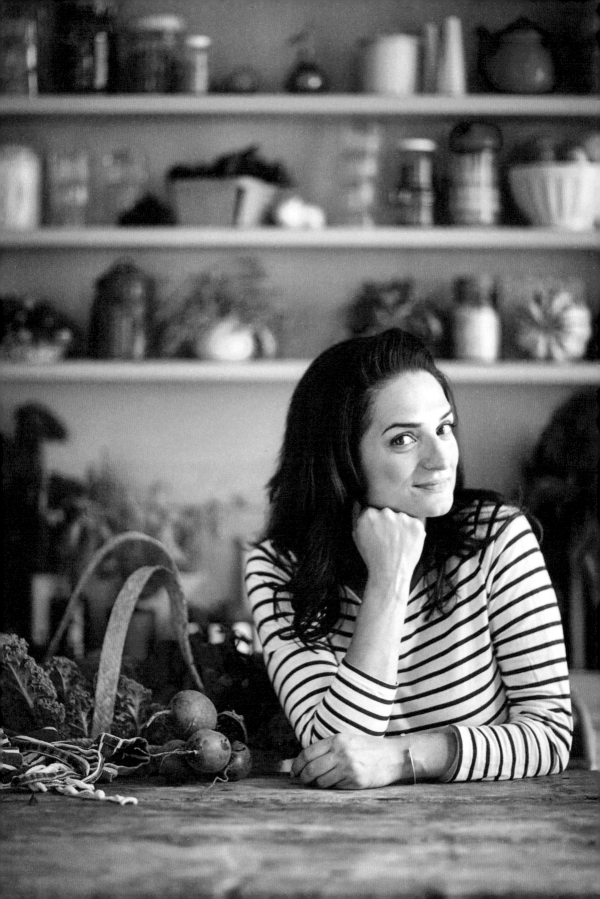

Introduction

~~~

So, here it is. At last! A book full of my favourite recipes for both fast days and feast days. Loads of delicious food that I hope you'll really get stuck into. Fresh, uncomplicated food. The book I really wanted to write.

It's for you, dear reader, and I hope you love it and use it and scribble on the pages and splatter it with food and lend it to your mates (who will then obvs buy a copy, too).

I think it was worth the wait. I hope you agree. Thanks for holding on so patiently.

Let's cook!

I love to see what people are cooking from the book so do post a photo of your creations online and tag me!

⊕ ellypear.com   🐦 @pearcafe
📷 @ellypear   f facebook.com/ellypearfood

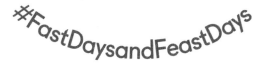

#FastDaysandFeastDays

Why I Started the 5:2

Surprise, surprise. I'm not a doctor. I can't advise you, but I can tell you what happened to me. My weight-loss story isn't complicated. I got fat because I ate too much food. I started the 5:2 and I lost the flab. That's it. In a nutshell.

OK, so there's a bit more detail you might be interested in. Five years ago, at 30 years old, I was bigger than I'd ever been. My weight had crept up and up and up. My boyfriend at the time (Dan) and I both had lives that revolved around food. We worked in the industry and our social life pretty much centred on eating. At that time I think we went to see a film ... once. We were both also pretty competitive and greedy and the combination led to us ordering and cooking way more food than we should.

I'd never tried any other sort of plan. I'm not the sort of person who goes from one diet to another, cutting out whole food groups and demonising certain ingredients while hero-worshipping others. A diet that meant I couldn't eat the things I wanted, or one that necessitated scrutinising menus to find something suitable, was never going to fit into my lifestyle.

However, this gluttony was making me fatter and fatter. Nothing fitted me any more and I was wearing about five per cent of my wardrobe. Even newer, larger-sized jeans would leave tight red marks around my waist at the end of the day. Not to mention I was feeling awful. I suffered from severe acid reflux (I couldn't bend over without feeling like I was going to vom) and my feet and knees were hurting from bearing the extra weight.

Dan had ballooned, too, and we were both well aware something needed to change. Dan started running and stopped ordering a spare main course (for real) and the weight dropped off.

I live an active lifestyle. I stand up all day for work (and always have done), I walk and cycle everywhere – and although I don't often do any extra exercise, I knew that no amount of sport could counterbalance the amount I was eating. As Jillian Michaels (the badass TV trainer) always says, you can eat your way through any amount of exercise. For me, the answer was clear. I had to put the reins on my eating habits.

During this same period, two friends in Bristol had started the '5:2 diet'. Like many people, I'd heard of it and had watched Michael Mosley's brilliant *Horizon* documentary, *Eat Fast and Live*

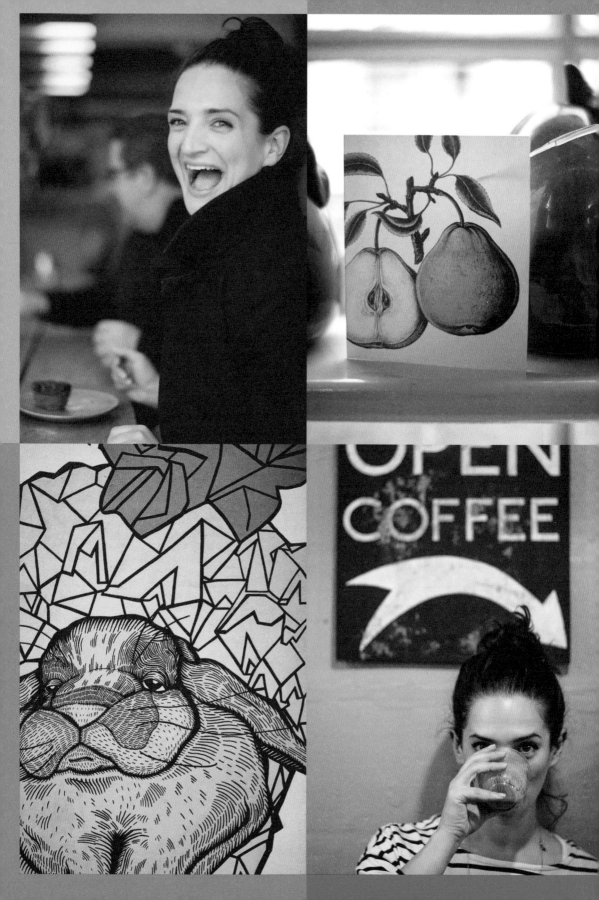

Longer. These two mates of mine both work in food as journalists for national papers, and their eating commitments are seriously demanding. There's not often a day where they don't have to be at a tasting, reviewing a restaurant or working on a recipe. I witnessed them both have huge success with the 5:2 and I reckoned this might just be the answer.

The thing that really grabbed me about the diet was that five days a week I could carry on as normal, eat what I liked, go out for dinner, work on recipes, and I just had to be careful on two days of the week. I loved the new challenges in the kitchen that fast days posed. The decision to cook fresh food from scratch while ensuring my meals were low-cal on these days was never really a decision; it was an obvious choice. I wasn't prepared to let go of everything I cared about and start eating packaged diet foods, just to keep within my calorie limits.

Right from the start, I used Instagram as a central part of my 5:2 experience. I posted what I'd made and tagged it #ellypearfastdays. I enjoyed showcasing my new ideas (aka showing off) and I was fascinated by people's comments. In all honesty, reading them kept me focused and stopped me from giving up because I felt like there was an audience waiting to see what I'd made.

The rules of the 5:2 as I saw them are very straightforward. Read Dr Mosley's book for a thorough understanding of the science involved. I'm here to show you the best way to use your calorie allocation. I can help you make a fast day something you'll enjoy, full of delicious food rather than a sad, grey day featuring a horrible line-up of unsatisfying packaged diet foods.

On two days a week I am very strict and eat up to 500 calories per day, never over.

The other five days a week, I eat whatever I like. I cannot stress this enough, but I will repeat it. On the other five days I eat whatever I like. That means no counting of calories, ever, no diary keeping, no worrying about anything. I simply eat a varied diet and try to stop eating when I'm full. If I want seconds, I have them. If I want to eat a whole pizza, I do. If I want to go out for dinner and order whatever I want, I do.

I view the seven days as a whole, with regards to nutrition. Within 500 calories, on any given fast day, it's incredibly hard to get all the protein, fats, carbohydrates, vitamins and minerals you need, so I make sure that on feast days I'm eating a good, balanced diet.

I'm a pescetarian (I eat fish, but not meat) and this is reflected in the recipes in this book, too. My diet is very heavy on veg and I do keep tabs to make sure I'm eating enough. In the UK, current government guidance states we should be aiming for five portions of veg and two of fruit a day (a recent increase from the five-a-day mantra). The total weight of these portions should equal at least 600g and nutrient-rich leafy greens should feature as much as possible. Considering that they contain most of their vitamins uncooked, it's a good idea to make sure you eat a healthy balance of raw vegetables. And it's a good idea to eat the peel of as much fruit and veg as possible (obviously not bananas and oranges!), as the majority of nutrients are concentrated near the surface.

Try to drink plenty of water on fast days – more than the eight glasses a day that are recommended – as the reduced amount of food you'll be eating means you'll be taking in less liquid in the form of food. Keep a jug of filtered water in the fridge and you'll find the water tastes better – plus, this way it's much easier to keep tabs on how much you're drinking.

Storecupboard Essentials

~~~

If your storecupboard is well stocked with the basics, then even a quick dash to the shops for fresh veg will result in a great dinner.

Dry goods

Oils – extra-virgin olive, olive, argan, sunflower, vegetable or rapeseed and coconut.

Vinegars – balsamic, sherry, white wine, red wine, rice wine, fruit (blackberry is great), malt (for chips, obvs).

Other condiments – mayonnaise, Worcestershire sauce, Tabasco and hot sauce (I use Frank's).

Spices and dried herbs – ground cumin, coriander and turmeric, Turkish chilli flakes, cardamom pods, cumin seeds, cinnamon sticks, garam masala, curry powder, cayenne, black mustard seeds, English mustard powder, bay leaves, sweet smoked paprika, dried oregano and thyme, ground cinnamon and vanilla pods.

Nuts and seeds – pistachios, hazelnuts, flaked almonds, walnuts, poppy seeds, sumac, nigella seeds, sesame, pumpkin and sunflower seeds.

Salt and pepper – sea salt flakes and smoked sea salt flakes (I use Maldon), Halen Mon chipotle chilli salt.

Rice and pulses – short-grain brown rice, red, green and Puy lentils.

Pasta – linguine and fusilli are my favourites and I use the De Cecco dried variety that is widely available in supermarkets.

Tinned and jarred ingredients – chickpeas, tomatoes (cherry, plum and chopped), beans (butter and cannellini), sweetcorn, passata, creamed horseradish, anchovies in olive oil, pickled jalapeños and capers.

Rolled oats

Date syrup and runny honey

Mini meringues

Asian ingredients – miso, sesame oil, furikake (Japanese rice seasoning), noodles (straight-to-wok Udon and black rice), tofu (plain and firm), soy sauce, hoisin, Sriracha chilli sauce, seaweed nori sheets, miso soup and rice paper wrappers.

Middle Eastern ingredients – pomegranate molasses, dried rose petals, flatbreads, tahini.

Healthfood store ingredients – smoked and/or marinated tofu, fresh sprouted grains, alternative pastas and flours, buckwheat, quinoa, Marigold vegetable bouillon powder, oat milk and raw cacao powder.

Fresh basics

Milk
I always buy organic milk. It is better in so many ways, for you, the cows, the farmers and the planet (look at www. organicmilk.co.uk for loads of interesting info) and it only costs a few pence more a pint than non-organic milk. I truly believe it also tastes so much better. 100ml of semi-skimmed milk is 50 kcal, whereas the same amount of whole milk equals 65 kcal. In a mug of tea, you'll typically use 2 tablespoons (30ml), so the difference is four calories. Basically, what I'm saying is if you use whole milk and you love it, it can totally be part of a fast day. Just measure it carefully, as with everything.

Butter
If I can get organic butter, yoghurts and cottage cheese, I buy them. Top-quality butter tastes miles better and it's really worth spending the extra money.

Yoghurt
I use both natural yoghurt and Greek yoghurt regularly on feast days and fast days. Yoghurt is high in calcium and protein, which may make you feel fuller for longer, so it's a good fast-day addition to meals. Shop around, too, and test out the different brands to see which work for you – but always check the calorie counts, as they will vary.

Eggs
I would be absolutely lost without eggs. I eat eggs most days and make sure I never run out! Buy free-range and organic if you can. Happy chickens lay much nicer eggs. I love Burford Brown eggs from Clarence Court for their superior taste and almost neon-bright yolks.

Quail eggs in particular are brilliant on fast days, as they contain just 15 calories each.

Essential Equipment

Food processor

Vegetable peeler

Mini blender

Zester

Baking tray

Grater (fine and coarse)

Roasting tin – ceramic
(lasagne) dish

Small and large frying
pans (non-stick)

Loaf tin

Silicon spatula

Large mixing bowl

Slotted spoon

Whisk

Mandoline

Small, medium and large
saucepans (lidded)

Sharp chef's knife and
chopping board

Digital scales

Measuring spoons

Juicer

Salad spinner

Colander

Tupperware containers

Sieve

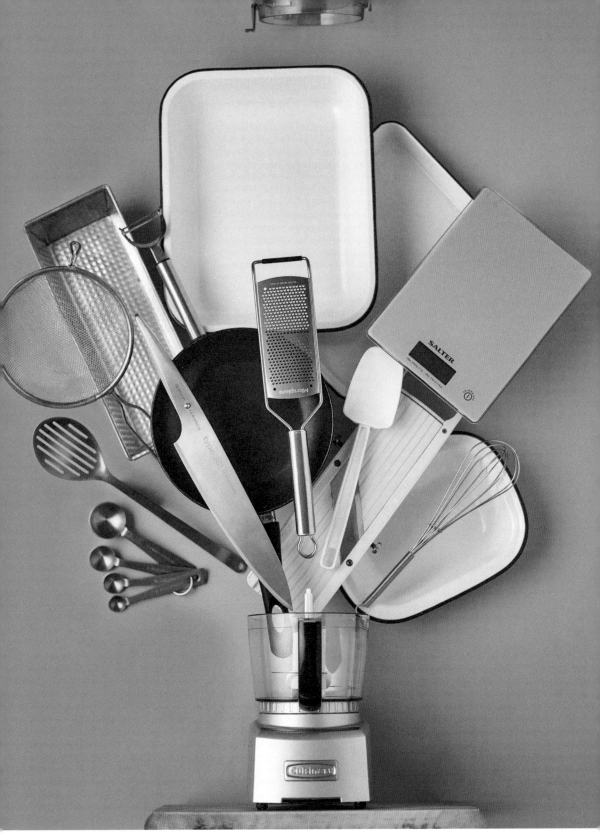

Essential Techniques

~~~

A few foolproof techniques that I rely on each week, for both fast and feast days

Cauliflower rice

There are loads of ways of making cauliflower rice and I've tried most of them. I don't have a microwave, so this is a quick and easy method made on the hob.

Cut the cauliflower into florets. Blitz the florets in a food processor until the size of breadcrumbs, using the pulse button. Tip into a dry, preheated non-stick pan, season well and cook, stirring continuously, over a medium heat with a rubber spatula until the cauliflower starts to catch and brown. Add a splash of hot water and cover with the lid (or foil). Turn the heat right down and allow the cauliflower to steam for 3–4 minutes, or until the water has evaporated. Turn the heat off and keep the pan covered. When ready to serve, tip into a bowl and stir through a handful of finely chopped coriander, parsley or mint. Or all three.

For freezing: Once you've got the food processor out to make the cauliflower rice, you might as well make more for the future and freeze it in portions. Get as many freezer bags ready as you want and weigh out 100g raw cauliflower rice into each, then seal. These are 34 calories each and can be frozen as they are (try to freeze them flat, with the cauliflower rice spread out in a thin layer). You'll need to defrost the cauli rice before you cook it, but that doesn't take long. Even if the rice is still a little bit icy, you can cook it from semi-frozen using the method above. You don't need to add hot water, just ensure that you heat it through so that it's piping hot.

6-minute egg

I like to cook my eggs using the 6-minute egg method, which gives a set white with a semi-runny yolk – creating a sort of dressing when broken into. These are excellent atop salads and dahls or soups. Make sure your egg is at room temperature before you cook it. Bring a small saucepan of water to the boil. Gently lower your egg into the hot water. Cook for 6 minutes, then remove the pan from the heat and pour away the hot water, holding your egg back with a spoon. Sit the (now dry) pan in the sink and turn the cold tap on, blasting the egg until it is cool enough to handle. Roll the egg on the counter, pressing down gently, until the shell cracks all over. Peel very carefully and serve on top of salad or whatever you like.

For a soft-boiled egg to eat out of the shell with soldiers, follow the above method but boil for just 5 minutes instead, and run under cold water for 5 seconds only, to stop the egg from cooking. Don't worry, this won't make your egg cold. Serve in an egg cup.

Courgette ribbons

You don't need a spiraliser, just use a vegetable peeler to make ribbons of raw courgette. Wash the courgette, then run the peeler down it lengthways, going over each section two or three times before rotating it and attacking a new section. Stop when you get to the seedy core. Do not throw this away; chop it up and chuck it in a soup or frittata or whatever is nearby.

You can also use a zester to make 'courgetti' using the same technique.

Kale

Kale is my absolute favourite veg. I've only been sick once this last winter and I've only gone a single week without eating kale. Both happened at the same time. Coincidence? I think not. Anyway. Try not to buy the 'prepped' bags of kale. They are not prepared well, generally, and usually contain lots of bits of tough stalk. It's this that tends to put people off. Buy a bunch of kale, if you can, take a big leaf in one hand, holding the main stalk, and simply pull the curly leafy bits off, working your way up the stalk. You'll end up with a pile of roughly torn kale and a bare, naked, tough stalk in your hand. Get rid of the stalk and wash the pile of leaves. Dry, but not too well. Heat a tiny (measured on a fast day!) bit of oil in a wok or large frying pan over a medium heat and chuck in the damp kale. Season well and stir continuously until wilted, about 5 minutes. Turn off the heat and

cover. This fry–steam method keeps the calories down, but results in a much nicer texture and flavour than simply steaming. Season well – sea salt and black pepper are essential. Lemon zest, chilli flakes and cumin seeds are all nice optional extras, too.

Rice

'Follow the packet instructions' is sod-all use if you buy rice in bulk by the scoop without a pack or label. I like to use short-grain brown rice (it's better for you and I prefer the nutty taste) and this is how I cook it.

For two very generous portions (one regular mug makes approximately 475g cooked rice): Boil a kettle of water. Fill a mug with brown rice and tip it into a sieve. Run the cold tap hard through the rice for about 30 seconds and shake so that the rice is thoroughly wet. Tip into a saucepan and add a big pinch of sea salt. Add two mugfuls of boiling water and stir well. Bring to the boil over a high heat, reduce the heat to low, cover, and simmer for about 20 minutes. Taste a few grains to check if it's cooked; the rice should be tender yet still have some bite. Depending on what kind of rice you are using, it may need a few more minutes. When it's cooked, take off the heat, drain in a sieve and then tip it back into the pan and repeat so that it is really well drained.

If you want to save leftover rice to eat the next day, you must do the following to avoid food poisoning. Cool the leftover rice down as quickly as possible (the easiest way to do this is to take it out of the pan, put it into a sieve and run cold water through it until it's totally cold). Then transfer the cooled, drained rice to a sealable tub and put it straight into the fridge, where it will keep for up to 48 hours.

Using storage containers to make your life better

It has only been in the last few years that I've really embraced this and I am pretty evangelical about it now. When Dan and I were running the supper club, we were eating more Chinese takeaways than is strictly necessary. After cooking solidly for days on end, we'd all too often reach for the phone and almost hug the delivery guy when he arrived. We started hoarding the plastic lidded containers to use to preserve stock in perfect 500ml portions that fitted snugly in our freezer, then we discovered loads of other uses for them. Matching tubs stack perfectly, which means your fridge space is used ultra-efficiently. We started running our home fridge more like our work fridges and the time, money and food savings that followed were substantial.

When you've finished plating up your dinner, transfer any leftovers to a tub (or tubs) and leave on the side (uncovered) while you eat. They will cool down and you can label and transfer them straight to the freezer once you've finished eating. I find this also helps to curb my tendency to help myself to seconds and thirds of something that was meant to last more than one meal!

When you open packets of messy things like smoked fish, cooked beetroot or feta, transfer them to a tub and seal well; you'll stop their flavour tainting other foods in the fridge.

If you use half a tin of something (chickpeas, chopped tomatoes, baked beans, etc.), transfer the leftovers to a sealed tub. Exposure to the air means that the food can become contaminated through contact with the lining material of the tin.

In the case of chickpeas and pulses, tip the entire contents into a sieve and rinse well with water, even if you're only using half.

I decant packets of spices, seeds and dried herbs into tubs and label them. We do the same at the café, and my god does it speed things up when you're cooking! If you use the end of something, you put the labelled tub to one side then, when it's time to do an online order or head to your local shops, you've got a ready-made shopping list. How good is that?! The simple things that make life so much better and easier.

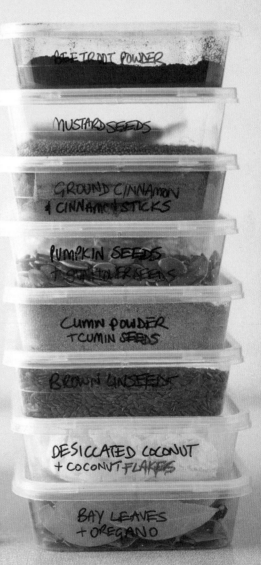

How I approach the greengrocers

I prefer shopping for veg at my local greengrocers rather than the supermarket. Buying just what you need rather than big packets of stuff means less packaging and less food waste. Eat fruit and veg in season as much as you can and visit the greengrocers regularly so you can see what's new each week. Don't feel embarrassed if you only need a tiny bit of something, like a single chilli, and if you're shopping just for yourself, don't be afraid to ask if they'll split things – my grocer will sell half a bunch of herbs and will even cut a cabbage or a watermelon in half if they're sure they can sell the second half – just do it politely.

Fresh produce

When you get home from the shops, invest a bit of time in washing and carefully storing your fruit and veg. Lay a folded sheet of kitchen paper in the base of your fridge drawers to absorb any moisture and you'll find that produce lasts much longer than usual.

The way we wash and store salad leaves at the café is a really golden trick that I'm going to share with you. Buy mixed bags of salad leaves from the supermarket and they'll turn to stinky slime very quickly – rarely lasting past two days. Do it the Pear Café way and your lettuce will last at least four days. Buying whole lettuces rather than prepped leaves will save you money, too.

We use oakleaf and little gem lettuce at the café, but the same technique works for any lettuce.

Fill your sink with ice-cold water. Cut the base off the lettuce, cut out the hardest section of core with the tip of your knife and separate the leaves.

Plunge the leaves into the cold water and swish them around with your hand. Transfer to a large bowl, drain the sink and refill with ice-cold water. Rinse the leaves a second time. Take a double handful of leaves and shake them as dry as you can over the sink. Move into a salad spinner and spin really well, pouring away the water every few seconds. The leaves must be totally dry before you continue. Lay a few sheets of kitchen paper inside the largest zip-lock bags you can find. Keeping the leaves whole (cut edges will turn brown quickly), fill the zip-lock bags up to the top, but don't overfill them. Gently lay the bags flat in the bottom of your fridge (or the crisper drawer) and avoid putting anything on top. Change the kitchen paper every day if it looks wet.

Organising your week

'When do you do your fast days?' is one of the most commonly asked questions. It varies each week, and apart from ensuring I don't do two consecutive days (I'd go mental), I don't make any other rules. If you start each week on a Monday, if anything comes up and you need to postpone a planned fast day, you can find yourself careering towards the weekend still having to fit one in. For that reason, I split my weeks up from Thursday to Wednesday. I look at my diary and work out what commitments I need to work around. Obviously, dinners out or lunch meetings need to be accounted for. Also bear in mind what else you have on that week. I often do a Monday and a Wednesday, but do whatever is right for you. If you don't work Monday to Friday, nine to five, you might find that fitting one fast day on a weekend suits you better. Play around, but be firm with yourself and don't postpone a fast day unless you really have to.

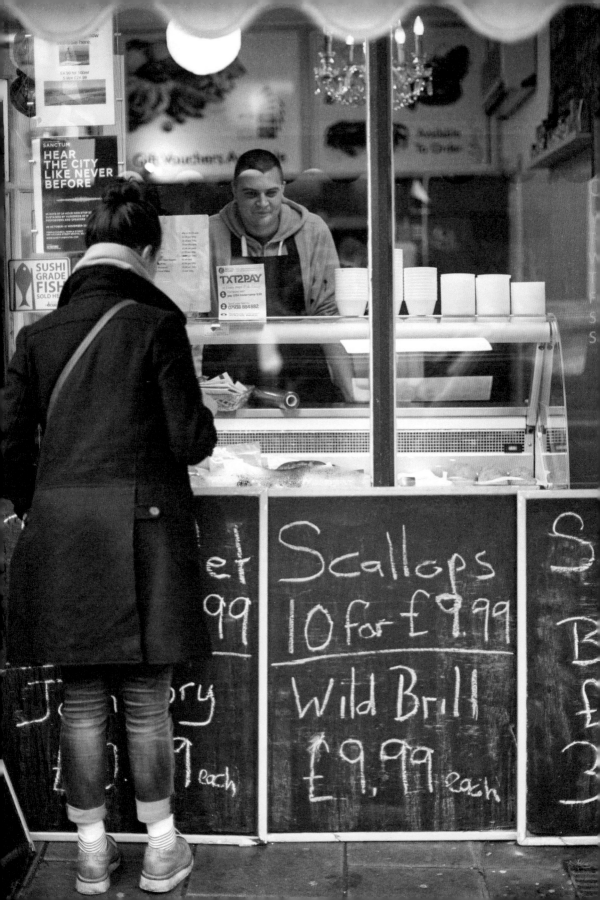

Leftovers

If you use leftovers cleverly, you will save so much money. I can't emphasise this enough. You'll also discover great new flavour combos as you get creative with random bits and you're obviously reducing food waste, too. I've suggested loads of ideas throughout the book of how you can use up any half-opened packets of things, but here are some more simple ones:

Nearly all the recipes in the Weeknight Dinners chapter can be chilled overnight and reheated at work the next day. Take a few fresh herbs and some crunchy toasted seeds to add that extra bit of texture.

Leftover dhal, warmed up for breakfast and topped with a fried egg, a drizzle of Sriracha and a soft chapatti, is a seriously delicious start to the day. Stir chopped avocado through a batch of Kachumber (see page 223) and add spoonfuls as a topping for dhal – this makes a great thing even better.

Leftover roast veg make a great vegetarian toad in the hole. Make up a batter in a large bowl with equal volumes of egg, self-raising flour and milk, season, add some finely chopped herbs, a heaped tablespoon of creamed horseradish (or a teaspoon of English mustard powder), whisk well, pour into a large jug and leave to sit for half an hour. The batter should be the consistency of double cream. Splash some oil in a small baking tin and put it into a preheated oven at 220°C/425°F/Gas mark 7 until it starts to smoke. Add the cooked veg and toss. Put back in the oven for 5 minutes, then pour the batter over and around the veg into the hot tin. Return the tin to the oven and cook for 20 minutes until the batter mixture is puffed up and golden brown.

Remember, pretty much any leftovers can be made into a frittata (aka a fridgetatta!), or add a 6-minute egg (see page 16) or a fried egg to jazz up your leftovers. This can often stretch dinner for one into dinner for two, for just a few pence.

The freezer is only one way to preserve things. Don't forget about pickling, making chutneys and jams, etc. The Marinated Feta on page 231 is a great example.

Make a soup. Chuck in any veg (cooked or raw), along with some herbs (even sad old limp bits), a tin of chickpeas or some lentils and top up with stock. Blitz and what was once destined for the bin has found a whole new life.

Social eating – when you and the people you're eating with want different things

On many of the fast-day recipes, you'll find feast-day upgrades or quick and easy ideas to transform that fast-day recipe into a feast-day recipe. If you're a woman (who is keeping under 500 kcal on a fast day) cooking with a man who is also on the 5:2 and is allowed 600 kcal, then feast-day upgrades could be useful for the additional 100 kcal. If you're making a meal for a non-faster, add the upgrade with wild abandon! One example is the Lentil and Red Pepper Chilli (see page 102), 271 kcal per portion. To add 100 kcal, serve sprinkled with 25g grated Cheddar or 35g crumbled feta.

To make a #feastdayupgrade, serve with sliced avocado, soured cream and brown rice.

To satisfy meat eaters, fry off some little cubes of chorizo and stir through the chilli as you reheat it. Or make some skewers of grilled chicken.

How and Where I Shop

~~~

I'm really lucky to live where I do and be able to shop the way I want to, I'm fully aware of that. Bristol is incredibly well provided for and I can get every ingredient in this book within walking distance.

I also know that not everybody has the same access to ingredients that I do, so here are some online resources for all the ingredients that you may have trouble finding. Having said this, the vast majority of the ingredients in this book can be found in even a small supermarket.

Shop in independent shops whenever you can and support small business owners. Give the money you're spending to the people feeding you, whenever you can.

Watch the seasons change and learn what is in season when by getting a veg box delivered or visiting your local greengrocer. Try new things and experiment, whenever you can.

Get your dry stores (tinned goods, rice, spices, oils, etc.) organised and do a check every once in a while so that you know when something is running out. Label them clearly. Any recipe that includes long lists of spices is infinitely more approachable (and economical to make) if you already have everything, and can find it, i.e. nothing goes to Narnia in the jumble at the back of your storecupboard.

Keep in mind that it's much cheaper to buy foods in bulk, so do a big shop for things like pulses and grains every few months and then you don't need to think about it for ages. You're also saving on time and packaging this way.

Buying tiny jars of things from the supermarket is crazy expensive. If you live in a city, head to an Asian supermarket and, for example, you'll get a huge bag of sesame seeds for half the price of a tiny jar from the supermarket. The same goes for big tubs of miso, bottles of Sriracha and soy sauce, tubes of wasabi and packets of noodles. Head to a Middle Eastern shop and you'll find bottles of pomegranate molasses, tubs of tahini, tinned chickpeas and bags of dried rose petals for bargain prices. Polish shops have an abundance of pickled foods that add zing to any meal and Korean shops will (of course) sort you right out for gochujang (fermented chilli paste) and kimchi. Discovering new ingredients and integrating them into my cooking is one of my greatest pleasures, and experimenting is the best way to learn. Chat to the shop owners, as sometimes they'll give you new ideas and sometimes you'll surprise them with your plans! My local Indian suppliers would quiz me on what I did with the huge sacks of nigella seeds I was always buying from them. I told them I'd sprinkle nigella seeds over salads and put them into soups – this was a novel idea to them, as they'd only ever used them in Indian dishes. Same goes for the Korean shop owner who reacted with a giggle when I told her that I spread miso paste on my toast. There are no rules to what you can do with the things you've bought. Go for it. It's your dinner.

Online resources

If you can't get to shops like these, I can't recommend www.souschef.co.uk highly enough. Their range covers Middle Eastern and Asian staples, as well as all the grains, herbs and spices you'll ever need. They also stock tableware, equipment and odd kitchen bits, too, like disposable piping bags. And their prices are very reasonable. Also have a look at the following sites for all sorts of goodies …

www.foratasteofpersia.co.uk/shop
Particularly for Middle Eastern ingredients.

www.hollandandbarrett.com/shop/food-drink
For all sorts of speciality products such as Maca powder, but not the chilled items like tofu that they stock in their high-street shops.

www.goodnessdirect.co.uk
An online healthfood shop with a notably impressive range of tofu.

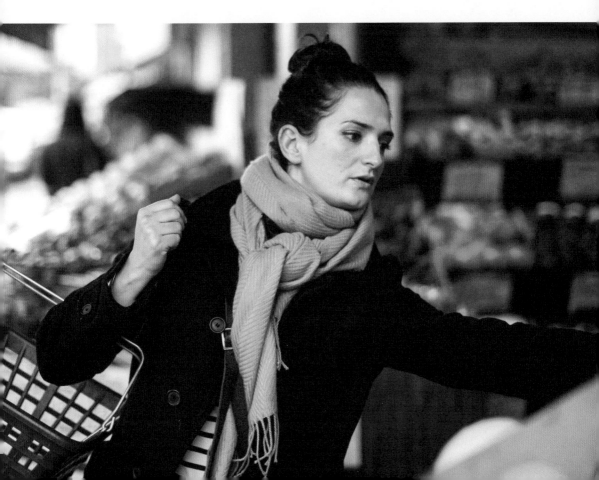

Fast-Day Drinks

~~~~~

Be very careful – drinks count as calories too. It might seem obvious to say that, but I speak to people all the time who 'don't count' tea and coffee. If you add milk, and especially sugar, your calories are mounting up quietly. Drink away from your own home, and you're in very little control of what you consume.

Obviously, going out to a café or bar to meet friends is something you don't want to stop doing if you're on a fast day, so here are my top tips.

Water

Drink loads. More than you think you need. Your skin will look better for starters. Add fresh mint or lemon or cucumber or slices of root ginger to a big jug and keep it in the fridge. Tap water tastes better filtered and chilled – fact. Apparently, it's easier for your body to absorb warm water than cold, though, so include at least a couple of mugs of boiled (then cooled) water each day too. And obviously it's zero calories. Still, fizzy, cold, hot; it's all zero.

Tea and coffee

The lowest-calorie option is to drink tea or coffee without any milk or sugar added.

There are LOADS of delicious teas out there with minimal calorie counts that you should try.

I'm not a fan of fruit tea and would much rather go for a jasmine, Earl Grey, green or mint tea. Experiment with multiple infusions (i.e. use the leaves more than once to brew cup after cup) and what might seem like an expensive investment could become a rather frugal highlight to your fast day.

The rise of good coffee in this country is a good thing all round. Avoid chain coffee shops at all costs (as an independent café owner, I would say that, wouldn't I?!) and head to a small independent who knows what they're doing and is passionate about their product.

Developments in the way in which coffee is brewed means that a beautifully clean, light coffee emerges from brew methods like the Aeropress or V60. I drink these straight black. One cup equals between 4 and 8 calories, depending on the size. I try to avoid drinking too much coffee on an empty stomach, though, as it can leave you feeling really wired and weird. One cup, however, can give you a boost mid-afternoon. I'll have a mug of builder's tea first thing, measuring the milk carefully. The rest of the day, I'll drink water or calorie-free teas, and a coffee mid-afternoon. Adding sugar to tea and coffee is a habit that's understandably hard to break, but if you can do it, you're saving yourself hundreds of calories over a week. Drink just three cups of tea per day, with two sugars in each, and that's 630 kcal a week.

Booze

Can you drink alcohol on a fast day? It's a good question, and one that I get asked a lot.

As mentioned, the 500 kcal a day rule can be interpreted any way you like. That said, using up your 500 kcal on alcohol alone would make you a crazy person (and drunk).

On a fast day, drinking alcohol will affect you more than you're used to; it'll absorb into your blood stream quicker. Here are some options for alcohol so that you can still join your mates for a drink on fast days. Have just one, then switch to fizzy water with fresh lime. It'll look like a G&T.

A pint of wine This started as a joke, and obviously is absolutely NOT a pint of wine. What it is is a very weak spritzer. If I'm with friends who are drinking pints, drinking one tiny glass of wine means I'll be finished before they are. So, what I started doing was ordering a 125ml glass of dry white wine (FYI, all pubs and bars have to be able to serve this size, even if it's not listed on the menu) and asking the bar staff to tip it into a pint glass, topped up with lots of ice and soda water. It lasts for ages (it's a pint of wine!) but is only 100 kcal.

A glass of fino sherry is my absolute favourite. 50ml is 50 kcal. The only issue being that it goes so brilliantly with salty fried snacks, which are not exactly a great #fastdayidea.

A glass of champagne (served in a 125ml flute) is approximately 100 kcal, depending on the brand. As a general rule, the drier the champagne, the lower the calories.

Vodka + lime + soda not using lime cordial, but just 2 freshly squeezed wedges of lime. A single shot of vodka, topped up with soda and two wedges worth of lime juice, is 67 kcal.

Half a pint of lager Approximately 115 kcal, depending on the brand.

The other option, of course, is not to drink alcohol at all. I don't mean all week, don't worry! However, having a few totally alcohol-free days during the week is very wise and will give your body a rest – you could use your fast days to have two at least. Bear in mind that cutting down on booze is often a huge factor for a lot of people's weight loss. Less alcohol leads to fewer hungover bad food choices and late-night unhealthy binges.

FAQs

~~~~

You've probably got a lot of questions at this point. I think the best way to cover as much ground as possible is to answer some of them with this list of questions I am often asked about the 5:2 concept.

Can you really eat what you want on feast days?

I wish I could include a clip here of the scientist who first introduced Michael Mosley to the concept of the 5:2. She clearly states you can eat 'whatever you like' on the five days. Just make sure it follows your regular eating pattern.

500 calories is nothing? Aren't you starving all the time?

No, I'm not. It's all about choosing the right things so that you can eat plenty of low-calorie foods and not feel deprived.

How do you work out your calories?

I use digital scales and measuring spoons to weigh and measure everything carefully and then use an app on my phone called 'MyFitnessPal' to input all the info. All the calories have been worked out for you in the fast-day recipes, but they're only accurate if you stick exactly to the recipe. Change any element, even by a few grams, and the calorie count will be wrong. Also, brands vary in their calorie counts. You should be recording every single thing you eat on a fast day and inputting the calories to ensure you do not go over 500 (for women) or 600 (for men). (This is based on the average person doing light exercise. If you do more intense activity, you will need more. The Michael Mosley website (www.michaelmosley.co.uk) has a great calculator for this.) If you are following one of the fast-day recipes from this book, you can simply note the calories for the recipe as a whole and add in the rest of the food for that day individually. I've carried on eating whatever I like on feast days.

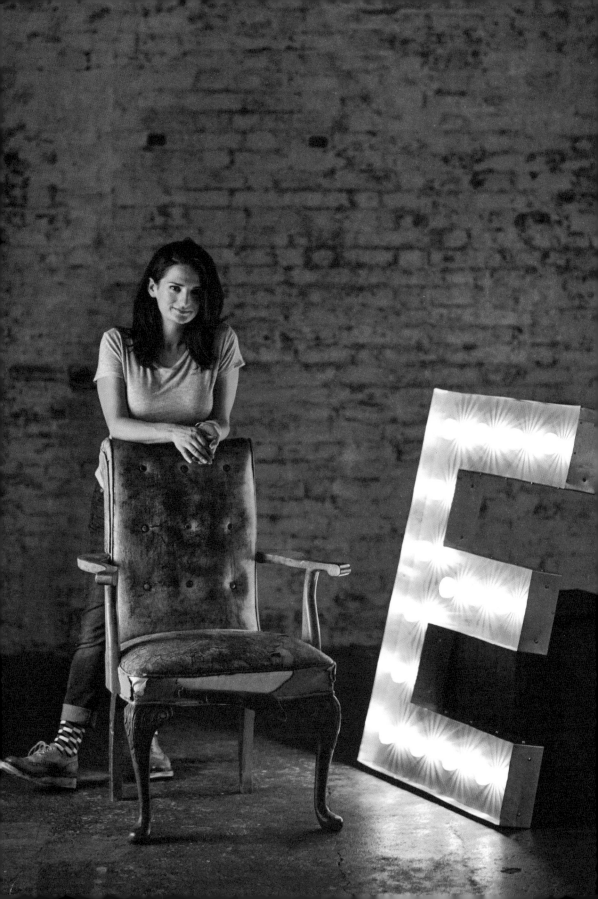

What time of day is best to eat?

The answer to this varies for everyone. When you start the 5:2, it's quite hard to predict when you're going to be hungry. You may coast through until lunchtime not hungry at all and then be hit by a massive slump in the afternoon and need to eat straight away, or you may find that eating early stops you feeling hungry all day. The 100-calorie lunch boxes on page 76 are designed for this very situation. Make up four of these boxes on your first fast day, leaving 100 calories for drinks and snacks.

How can I control my moods?

This is a tricky one. Having supportive people around you is the key to success here. There is no doubt that you're bound to have a bit of a short fuse at times, but preparation is crucial. The spikes of grouchiness tend to occur for me when I am in a shop, trying to decide what to make for a fast day, and feeling impatient. The hungry anger kicks in and I feel like I need to eat NOW. I'm always trying to come up with new recipes every fast day (it's kind of my job), so I have that added pressure. You don't need to feel that way. Get organised, have plenty of prepared nibbles and apologise if you're being grumpy. It'll be all better once you've eaten.

How often do you cheat?

Hand on heart, never. You have to develop quite a stubborn determination on fast days. Remember, it's only one day... When you wake up tomorrow, you can eat whatever you like.

What are your favourite high-satisfaction, low-calorie foods?

Protein is great for making you feel fuller for longer, but I get the most satisfaction on fast days from plenty of crunchy raw veg, with a controlled amount of toppings and dressings. What is definitely the least satisfying is deciding to use up calories on something like a single finger of a Kit-Kat, simply because you're craving chocolate. Just don't do it. It's not worth it and you'll only want more. Remind yourself that tomorrow you can have whatever you like.

How do you make the 5:2 work if you work shifts?

Not everybody works Monday to Friday, nine to five. Fitting in fast days when you're working shifts can sometimes take a little creativity. To explain my 'bridged fast' idea, you need to view a regular fast day not as 24 hours but as the (approximately) 34 hours it really is...

Here is an example of how the hours work out if you were doing a fast day on a Tuesday, presuming you stop eating/drinking by 10 pm the night before and start eating/drinking whatever you like at 7am the day afterwards:

Day	Times	Total Hours
Monday	7am–10pm FEASTING	
	10pm–7am FASTING	9
Tuesday	7am–10pm FASTING	15
	10pm–7am FASTING	9
Wednesday	7am–10pm FEASTING	

So, if you want to 'bridge' your fast over more than one day for whatever reason, you need to do 34 hours, not 24. You could do it as follows:

Breakfast meeting on Tuesday that you can't avoid: 8–10am – Eat whatever you like (feast), then start your 34-hour fast (500 calories) from after breakfast at 10am until 8pm on Wednesday. Like this:

Tues breakfast	FEAST (finish by 10am)
Tues lunch	FAST
Tues dinner	FAST
Weds breakfast	FAST
Weds lunch	FAST
Weds dinner	FEAST (eat after 8pm)

You're basically having one big meal and two smaller meals, two days in a row, which I think a lot of people would find more approachable.

NB: I've tried out this method at times when I've had unavoidable prior engagements and it worked well for me. Friends doing shift work or trying to fit fasting into challenging schedules have had success with it, too, but it has not had the same long-term testing that the 'traditional' format has.

Once I've done the 5:2, should I move on to 'maintenance mode'?

I started the 5:2 in April 2013 at 148lbs and after 5 months, I'd lost a stone. I carried on losing weight at a very steady pace and in January 2015 I moved to 'maintenance mode' – that is, 6:1. Although I've found that doing a single fast day a week is enough to maintain weight loss, it's definitely not the green ticket to eat what you like on feast days (unlike on the 5:2). On the 6:1 I actually found that I needed to be extra careful about what I ate on the six feast days. For that reason, I'm actually happier on the 5:2. It's up to you, though; by all means try it and see what works for you.

What about exercise and fasting?

I live an active lifestyle – I stand up all day for work and walk and cycle everywhere, but I rarely do intensive physical exercise. If you're exercising intensively, or in training, you may struggle with the 5:2 approach as you may not be able to refuel sufficiently on restricted calories. Common sense tells me that you should listen to your body. On fast days I sometimes feel like I could run up mountains (in Michael Mosely's original *Horizon* film, he went on a long walk on one of his first fast days – and survived) and if you're feeling up to it, crack on. But, similarly, if you're feeling in any way not up for it, don't push yourself. As I said, it's common sense. There are five other days in the week to get your sweat on.

Can I start the 5:2 with a history of an eating disorder?

If you have been diagnosed with an eating disorder now or in the past, do consult your GP or health practitioner before starting this approach.

Can I do the 5:2 while breastfeeding?

If you are pregnant or breastfeeding, do consult your GP or health practitioner before starting this approach.

I have coeliac disease. Can I do the 5:2?

Absolutely, in fact you'll find most of the recipes are gluten free.

What to eat on feast days

The whole point of the 5:2 is that you do not count calories on feast days. You will lose weight more slowly if you really overindulge on your feast days, but the whole point is to free yourself from restrictive diets for the majority of your week and only count calories on fast days. How do you not go OTT on the other five days? My advice would be, don't buy crap. Don't fill your cupboards with rubbish and you won't fill yourself with rubbish. If there are only healthy foods in your cupboards and fridge, the most 'indulgent' you can get is to have a massive portion of rice with your dinner or slosh olive oil all over your salad. Even so, neither of these things are bad. You're cooking from scratch, using fresh ingredients and after a fast day, things you might not have previously considered a treat really do feel like one. The 5:2 recalibrates your appetite and tastes in this way.

After a fast day, have a look in your fridge; you may find that there are more half-used and open packets than usual, as you've only needed, for example, half a pack of tofu or only a portion of smoked fish from the pack. Incorporate these leftover elements into your feast-day dinner. Think of what you had to painstakingly weigh out the day before and enjoy not having to measure or weigh anything. If you continue to take the lessons you've learnt on the fast days regarding cooking fresh food from scratch and carry them over to feast days, then you're already winning. 'Eating clean' has become an overused, almost meaningless phrase but, as far as I'm concerned, this is all it comes down to. Enjoy dairy, enjoy gluten, enjoy carbs – just cook proper, fresh food and eat as much veg as possible. Simple.

The mental health benefits of this approach are not to be understated. Freeing yourself from unneccessarily restrictive diets and enjoying food is key to happiness.

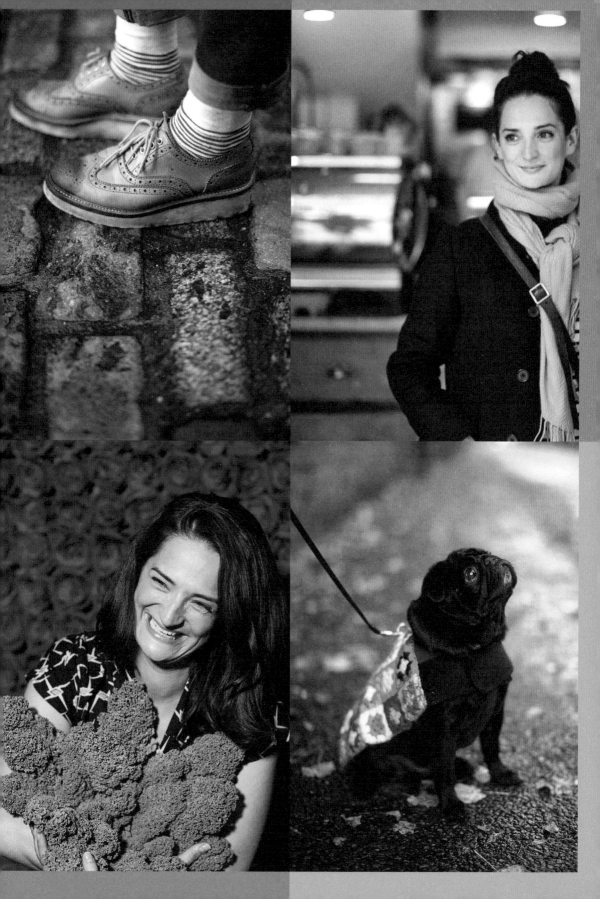

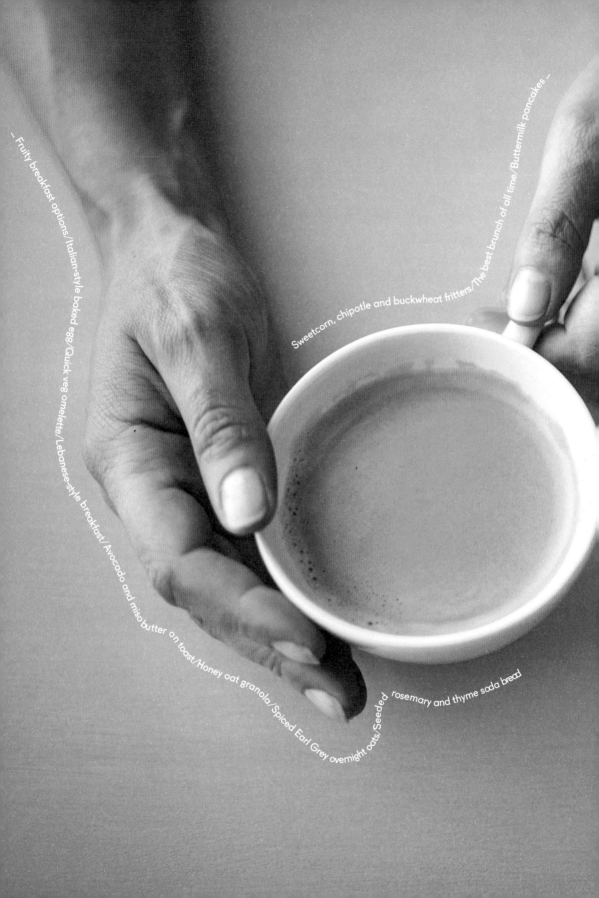

... Fruity breakfast options/Italian-style baked egg/Quick veg omelette/Lebanese-style breakfast/Avocado and miso butter on toast/Honey oat granola/Spiced Earl Grey overnight oats/Seeded rosemary and thyme soda bread

Sweetcorn, chipotle and buckwheat fritters/The best brunch of all time/Buttermilk pancakes ...

Breakfasts

and

Brunches

Seeded rosemary and thyme soda bread

This is THE bread to make if it's your first attempt or you're short of time. No kneading. No waiting for it to prove. It takes less than ten minutes to make. Mix it up like a cake mix, then whack it in the oven. Easy. It is unbelievable eaten straight out of the oven, but if kept wrapped tightly in a cotton tea towel it will be fine for a few days. It is better toasted after a couple of days, though.

This recipe makes a dense, seeded loaf that is incredibly filling, so one slice is usually enough. Usually.

Makes 1 loaf
(approximately 16 slices)
___

225g plain flour

225g wholemeal flour

1 heaped tsp bicarbonate of soda

1 heaped tsp cream of tartar

2 tbsp soft brown sugar

1 tbsp sunflower seeds

1 tbsp poppy seeds

1 tbsp sesame seeds

1 tbsp finely chopped rosemary

1 tbsp finely chopped thyme leaves

20g roughly chopped walnuts

1 tsp flaked sea salt

500ml buttermilk, or whole milk plus 1 tbsp lemon juice, or 250ml whole milk plus 125ml natural yoghurt left for 5 minutes

30g butter, melted

For the topping

1 tsp pumpkin seeds

2 tsp chopped rosemary

flaked sea salt

Preheat the oven to 200°C/400°F/Gas mark 6.

Sift the flours into a large bowl and tip in anything that remains in the sieve (you're just aerating the flour, not trying to remove all the wholemeal bits). Add the remaining dry ingredients, except for the toppings, and stir to combine.

Make a well in the centre of the dry mix and slowly pour in the buttermilk, mixing gently but thoroughly. It will form a loose, cake-type batter, not a bready type of dough – don't worry!

Brush a 10 x 20cm loaf tin with the melted butter. Put the mixture into the tin and even out the top using a spatula. Pour the remaining butter over the surface of the dough. Sprinkle with the toppings and bake for 30 minutes. Reduce the temperature of the oven to 150°C/300°F/Gas mark 2 and turn the loaf around. Bake for another 25–30 minutes, until a sharp knife inserted into the centre comes out clean.

Turn the loaf out onto a wire rack to cool slightly before eating. You can also let the bread cool completely, cut it up into slices, freeze, then toast from frozen.

Spiced Earl Grey overnight oats

The very best thing about this recipe is that if you spend a couple of minutes in the evening putting it together, in the morning you can just grab it out of the fridge and go. On a busy morning when the to-do list is as long as my arm, having instant breakfast ready to dip into whenever I have a minute between tasks is a godsend. Feel free to play around with fresh or dried fruits, different milks and yoghurts, seeds and nuts. There are no rules.

Serves 1
—

30g oats

1 Earl Grey tea bag

1 tbsp linseeds (flaxseed)

1 tbsp raisins

bit of cinnamon stick

1 clove

1 cardamom pod, crushed

1 tbsp desiccated coconut

70ml milk (any type, including nut milks)

Topping ideas

Greek yoghurt

fresh fruit or berries of choice

maple syrup

toasted coconut flakes

Put the oats in a jar, add the tea bag, the linseeds, raisins, cinnamon, clove, cardamom and desiccated coconut. Pour in the milk and about 125ml boiling water, just to enough to cover the oats. Give it a mix with a spoon, then put the lid on the jar. Tip the jar over a couple of times to combine all the ingredients and put it in the fridge overnight.

In the morning, top the oats with yoghurt, fresh fruit or berries, maple syrup, toasted coconut flakes and whatever else you fancy.

F
E
A
S
T

Honey oat granola

Making a big jarful of granola is a really great idea. You know exactly what is in it (unlike packaged cereals) and you can add or leave out whatever you like. This recipe is full of delicious ingredients, many of which are often described as 'superfoods' for their nutrient-rich properties. This isn't false advertising, but they're all in there for their flavour and texture. Some of the ingredients are expensive, but remember that you can make loads of batches simply by buying more oats (which are really cheap). Also, it's fine to leave the 'superfoods' out if you want, and make a simpler version with just the first five ingredients. It'll still be fantastic.

Makes 6 generous portions
—

200g honey

4 tbsp rapeseed or
    coconut oil

300g jumbo oats

50g whole almonds,
    very roughly chopped

3 tbsp raisins

1 tbsp raw cacao powder

1 tsp ground cinnamon

25g puffed buckwheat

2 tbsp pumpkin seeds

2 tbsp goji berries

2 tbsp hemp seeds

Preheat the oven to 200°C/400°F/Gas mark 6.

Melt the honey and rapeseed or coconut oil together in a large saucepan over low heat. Add the oats and almonds, and stir really well.

Take the mixture off the heat, spread it out on a large baking tray lined with baking parchment and bake for 17 minutes. Remove and leave to cool completely, then break up into chunks and put in a large bowl with the remaining ingredients.

Transfer to an airtight jar or Tupperware box and store in a cool, dry place for up to a month.

Serve with milk or yoghurt and top with any of your favourite fruit.

FEAST

145 kcal
per portion

Lebanese-
style
breakfast

This recipe was my friend Fiona Beckett's idea for a fast-day breakfast, and it has converted me to cottage cheese. In my mind, cottage cheese was linked with faddy Eighties' diets and aerobics, so I would always avoid it. But it's actually really nice and a lot lower in calories than other cheeses. It's full of protein, which helps to keep you feeling fuller for longer, too.

A perfect late breakfast or early lunch, this is also great for grazing on at your desk while you're at work. It is ideal for transporting in a lunchbox, too. Put the cheese or yoghurt in a little container or jar and everything else in a small box. On a feast day, add an extra toasted pitta and a few olives, or swap the pitta for olives if you need to avoid gluten.

F
A
S
T

Serves 1
—
50g cottage cheese

20g plain yoghurt

¼ tsp Za'atar (see page 228)

70g cucumber, cut into batons

50g tomatoes, cut into wedges

30g radishes, cut into wedges

1 mini pitta, toasted, or 15g black olives

Mix the cottage cheese with the yoghurt and put into a small serving bowl. Sprinkle with the za'atar and place on a plate, surrounded by all the other ingredients. Best served with black tea.

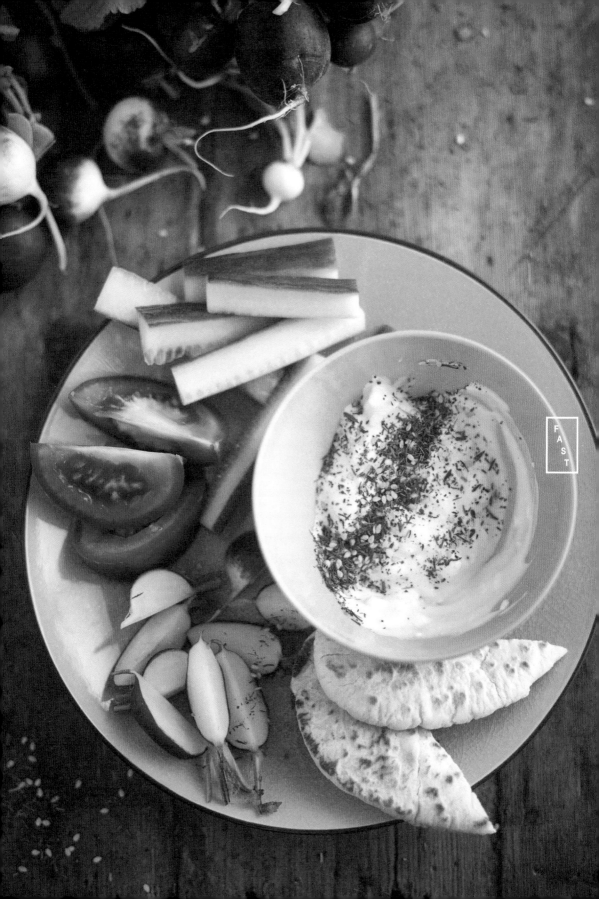

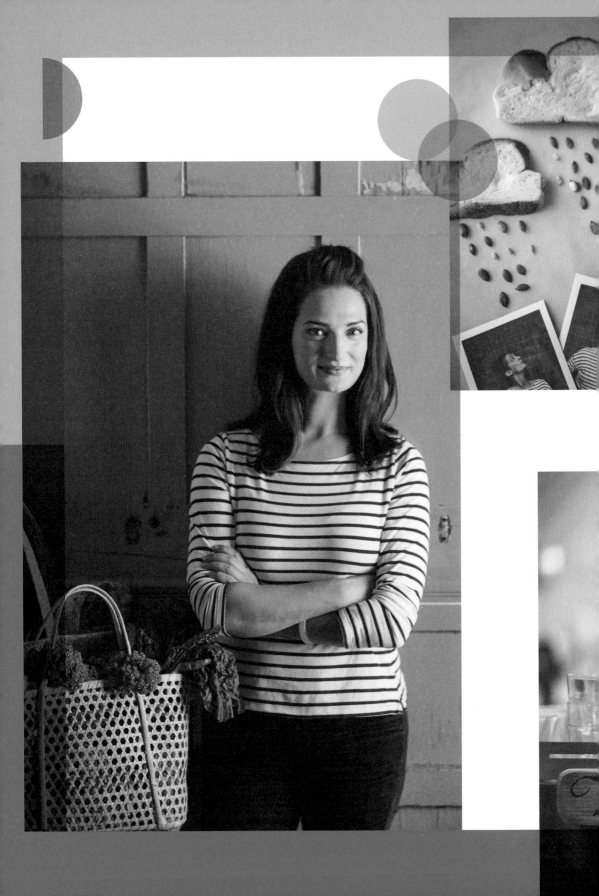

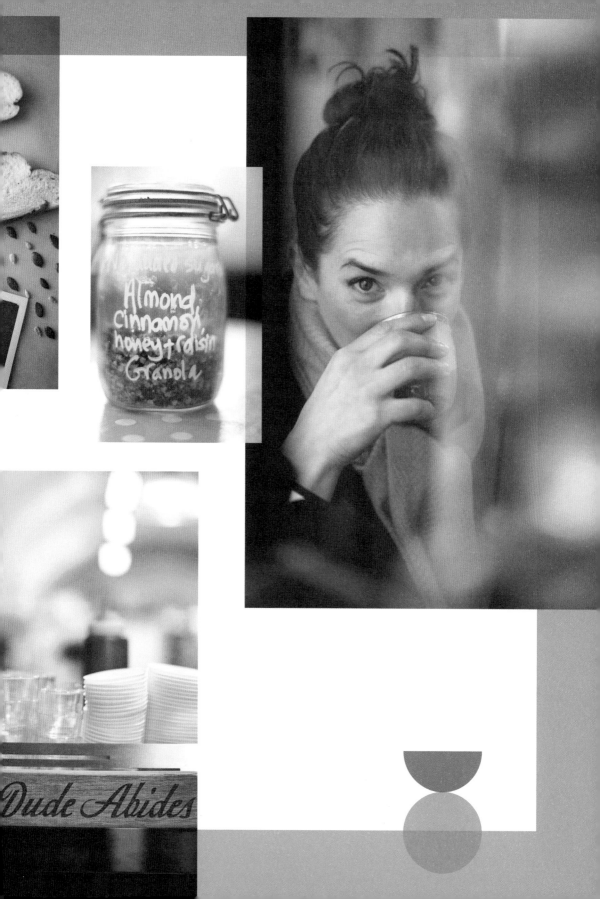

Quick veg omelette

If you can't even imagine starting a day without a proper breakfast, this is the fast-day recipe for you. You can make an egg-white-only omelette, but don"t: it will be gross!

Serves 1

20g cherry tomatoes, finely chopped

10g spring onions, finely sliced

30g chestnut mushrooms, sliced

1 egg

2g Parmesan, finely grated

1 tbsp finely chopped basil, chives or flat-leaf parsley

olive oil spray, for greasing

20g baby leaf spinach, finely chopped

flaked sea salt and freshly ground black pepper

The night before, mix the tomatoes, spring onions and mushrooms in a bowl. Cover and refrigerate overnight.

The next morning, break an egg into a jug, season well with salt and pepper and add the Parmesan, fresh herbs and 3 tablespoons water. Whisk well and set aside.

Spray the olive oil once on a 20cm non-stick frying pan and set over a medium heat. Add all the chopped refrigerated vegetables, season with salt and pepper, and cook for 10 minutes, until the mushrooms and tomatoes have started to brown.

Tip the vegetables back into their bowl, using a rubber spatula to make sure you thoroughly clear the pan.

Put the pan back over a medium heat. Tip in the egg mixture and swirl it around to cover the base of the pan. Pull the sides towards the centre and let the egg flow into the gaps you create. Tip all the cooked vegetables onto one side of the omelette and top with the baby spinach. Fold the omelette over, to encase the vegetables in a half-moon shape. The spinach will wilt in the heat. Serve.

Sweetcorn, chipotle and buckwheat fritters

These are best served as a weekend brunch with poached eggs and avocado and pico de gallo, or you could serve them for dinner sprinkled with feta and accompanied by a green salad, yoghurt and lime wedges.

Despite the name, buckwheat contains no wheat and it's not actually a cereal grain — it's a fruit seed that's related to rhubarb. It has a lovely nutty flavour. If you have other flours in your cupboard, try experimenting. This is a forgiving recipe; the flour is just there to bind, so lots of other flours would work easily. If you don't have any problems with gluten, you can of course use plain flour.

Makes 10 medium-sized fritters

300g sweetcorn kernels

4 spring onions, finely chopped

1 tsp chipotle chilli flakes

2 eggs

2 tbsp milk

120g buckwheat flour or plain flour, rice flour or polenta

olive oil

flaked sea salt and freshly ground black pepper

Mix the first six ingredients together well, then leave to rest for 5 minutes.

Heat the oil in a medium non-stick frying pan and shallow-fry large spoonfuls of the mixture over a medium heat, flipping when golden brown.

Drain on kitchen paper, sprinkle with sea salt and pepper and serve.

FEAST

Avocado and miso butter on toast

Using miso paste straight from the tub, like Marmite, was a bit of a revelation for me. I'd previously only used it dissolved into soups, but once I discovered how delicious it is blended with butter, I started using it on green veg and then on toast. I used to blend the miso and the butter together before realising that you can skip that step (that only creates more washing up) and spread it straight onto the toast! This is avocado toast taken to another level.

Serves 1

---

2 slices of good bread

¼ ripe avocado

2 tsp softened unsalted butter

1 tsp miso paste, or to taste

1 tbsp mixed sprouts

a few fresh coriander
    leaves, picked

1 tsp Pear Café Seed Blend
    (see page 227)

Sriracha sauce, to taste
    (optional)

Toast your bread.

Meanwhile, halve, destone and peel the avocado.

Using a sharp knife, slice the avocado lengthways into about 8–10 slices.

When the toast is done, butter it and then spread it with the miso, as if it's Marmite.

Lay the avocado slices on top and add the sprouts, coriander and seeds.

Add a splash of Sriracha if you want it spicy. Serve.

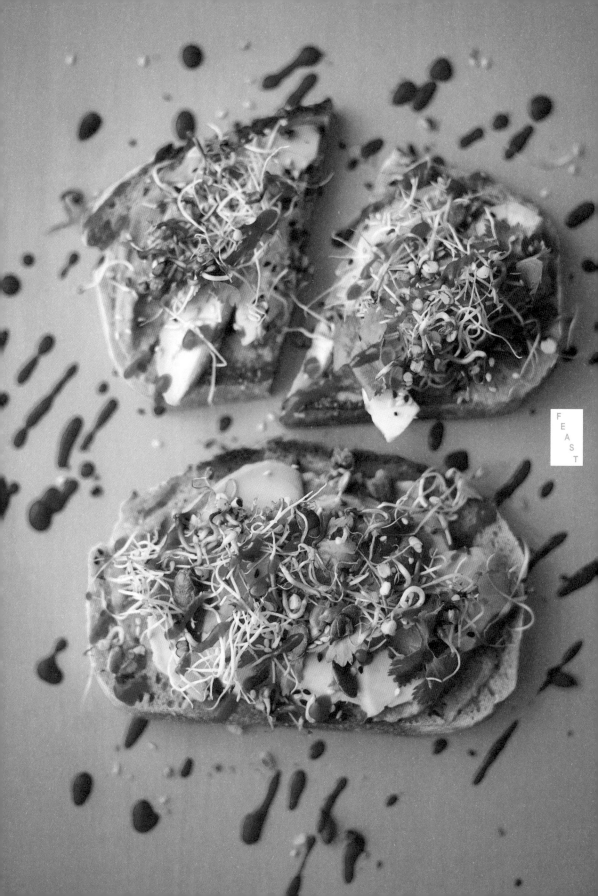

FEAST

Fruity breakfast
options

Chop up some fruit and mix together into a fruit salad or eat individually, with or without yoghurt. Remember when buying yoghurt to read the label and choose carefully. For the brands that I use low-fat natural yoghurt = 61 kcal per 100g, 0% Greek Yoghurt = 57 kcal per 100g.

Make it even better: squeeze over some fresh orange, lemon or lime juice and/or zest, add fresh mint, or sprinkle over some ground cinnamon or fresh vanilla seeds (make sure you account for whatever additions you make!). Nuts are a delicious addition, but measure them very carefully. Even one hazelnut, dry toasted and chopped up, is about 10 kcal (but totally worth it).

50g of the below fruit in calories

$\vee$

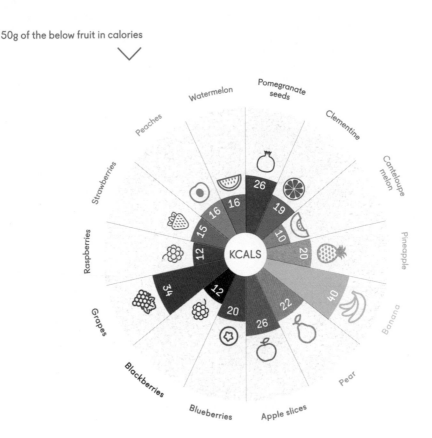

Buttermilk pancakes

These aren't crêpes, they're fluffy American-style pancakes. I think they're best not made too big and piled up in 3/4/5s. I eat mine with cold salted butter and maple syrup. My dad grew up in Canada and we always had maple syrup around the house when we were growing up. When I left home, I couldn't believe the price of the stuff. Treat yourself to a bottle and value it as the precious liquid gold it is.

Feel free to make amendments if you fancy. Add a few blueberries into the mix, sprinkling them on the surface of the pancakes just before you flip them over. Top with crème fraîche, sliced bananas and cinnamon, or serve with crispy bacon, if you're that way inclined.

Serves 2
—

For the dry mix

125g plain flour

1 tsp baking powder

¼ tsp bicarbonate of soda

¼ tsp salt

1 tbsp sugar

For the wet mix

1 free-range egg, beaten

375ml buttermilk, or whole milk plus 1 tbsp lemon juice, or 250ml whole milk plus 125ml natural yoghurt left for 5 minutes

2 tbsp melted butter, plus extra for frying

First, melt a large knob of butter in a frying pan and swirl it around. Pour 2 tablespoons of the melted butter into a jug and reserve the rest for greasing the pan. Add the remaining ingredients for the wet mix to the jug and combine.

Sift the dry ingredients together in a large bowl.

Make a well in the centre of the dry ingredients and pour in the wet mix.

Use a spatula to fold the two mixtures together gently (do not over-mix, you want some lumps remaining) and leave to sit, covered, in the fridge for 15 minutes to 1 hour.

When you're ready to eat, turn the oven on low and put a baking tray lined with baking parchment in there. This way, as you cook the pancakes you can slip them into the oven to keep warm.

Heat your frying pan over a medium heat. Fold a sheet of kitchen paper into a small square and dip it into the melted butter. Grease the frying pan with the butter.

Use a ladle to pour a puddle of mixture into the pan until it is approximately 10–12cm across. Leave the pan still and watch while bubbles start to emerge on the surface, then use your spatula to flip the pancake over. It should be golden brown. Cook on the other side until it's the same colour.

Eat straight away or pile up the pancakes in the oven (put sheets of parchment between them to prevent sticking) until they're all ready and everyone can sit down to eat together.

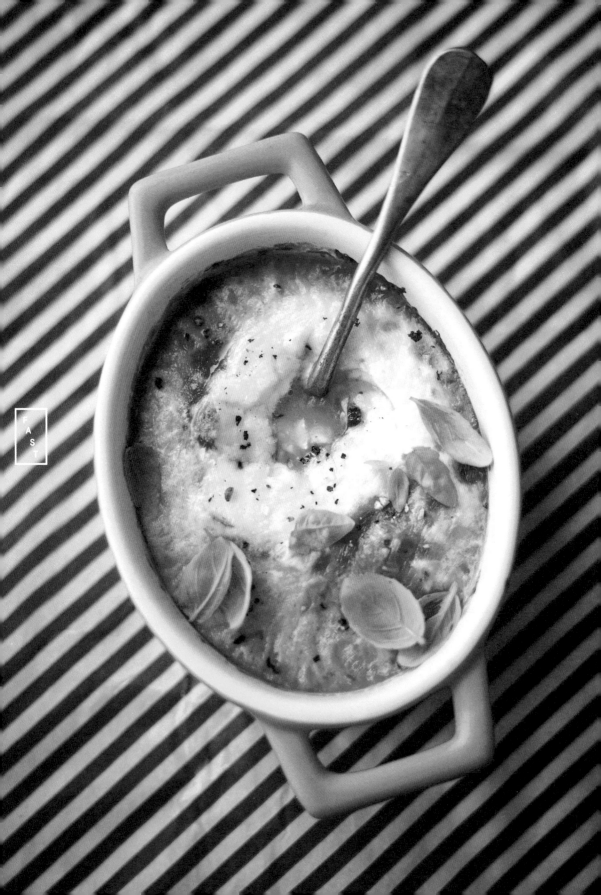

Italian-style baked egg

167 kcal
per portion

This recipe is so easy and so quick. It's a great filling breakfast but also a perfect weeknight supper or weekend brunch. I usually eat it with a teaspoon, on its own, and then make something else afterwards — maybe a big salad or some fish with vegetables. If you wanted something to dip into the egg and mop up the tomato juices with, a toasted mini wholemeal pitta is about 75 kcal (depending on the brand). Personally I'd rather use those 75 kcal up in the form of more veg or even a second egg in the dish itself. Adding roasted red peppers or wilted spinach or greens to the dish also works well. Add them to the saucepan along with the tinned tomatoes and use a bigger baking dish. Remember to adjust your calorie counts to allow for any amendments or additions.

Serves 1

¼ tsp olive oil

1 tsp finely chopped red chilli

1 garlic clove, crushed or very finely chopped

100g tinned cherry tomatoes

1 medium egg

2 tbsp semi-skimmed milk

5g Parmesan, finely grated

2 tbsp basil leaves (smaller leaves picked from a bunch)

flaked sea salt and freshly ground black pepper

Preheat the oven to 180°C/350°F/Gas mark 4.

Put the (very carefully measured) olive oil into a small saucepan and warm through. Add the chilli and garlic and cook over a low heat for about 4 minutes, being careful not to burn the garlic. Add the tomatoes and use the back of a spoon to gently crush them against the side of the pan, just to break them down a little. Stir well and continue to cook for a further 6 minutes. Tip the entire contents of the pan into a small ovenproof dish, making sure you scrape every last bit out (I used an oval dish approximately 10cm wide and 20cm long).

Crack the egg on top of the tomato mixture. Pour the milk on top of the egg, sprinkle over the cheese and season well with salt and black pepper. Bake for 10–12 minutes, until the egg white is set.

Remove from the oven and leave for a couple of minutes to cool. It tastes better once it's cooled down a tiny bit. Just before serving, sprinkle with basil leaves.

The best brunch of all time

If I had to choose one dish to eat for the rest of my life – for breakfast, lunch and supper – it would be this.

Satisfying, nutritious, it feels like a treat but also in no way unhealthy. All the textures and the pops of flavour really make this the queen of brunches.

I can't stress enough how important it is that you find the best produce you can. You're not doing much to any of the ingredients and the quality of what you put in will shine out of the finished dish.

This is for one person but if you're making it for 2, double everything (obvs) and get them to make the blooming tea.

Serves 1
—

1 egg, very fresh
1 tbsp white wine vinegar
1 slice of sourdough bread
2 big handfuls of kale
1 ripe avocado
glug of olive oil
2 tsp Pear Café Seed Blend
    (see page 227)
a few sprigs of coriander,
    leaves picked
Sriracha sauce, to taste
flaked sea salt and freshly
    ground black pepper

For the tea
tea bag
milk (optional)

Fill your kettle with water. Put your tea bag in a mug. Get everything out the fridge and lay it out on the benchtop.

Break your egg into a small cup or bowl.

Fill a medium-sized saucepan about a third full with boiling water from the kettle and add the vinegar. Put on the hob over a medium-high heat and let the water simmer while you prepare the other bits.

Put your bread into the toaster, but don't press it down yet.

Next, pull the kale leaves off their tough stalks and put in a colander. Rinse well under warm water and give them a good shake. You don't want them totally dry, don't worry.

Cut your avocado in half and twist to separate. Either peel the skin off or, starting at the narrow end, dig a spoon in, between the skin and the flesh, to free the flesh in one go. Reserve one half for later on and slice the flesh of the other half into 8–10 slices lengthways and put to one side.

From this point it's all going to come together quickly, so have a final check that everything is out and prepared.

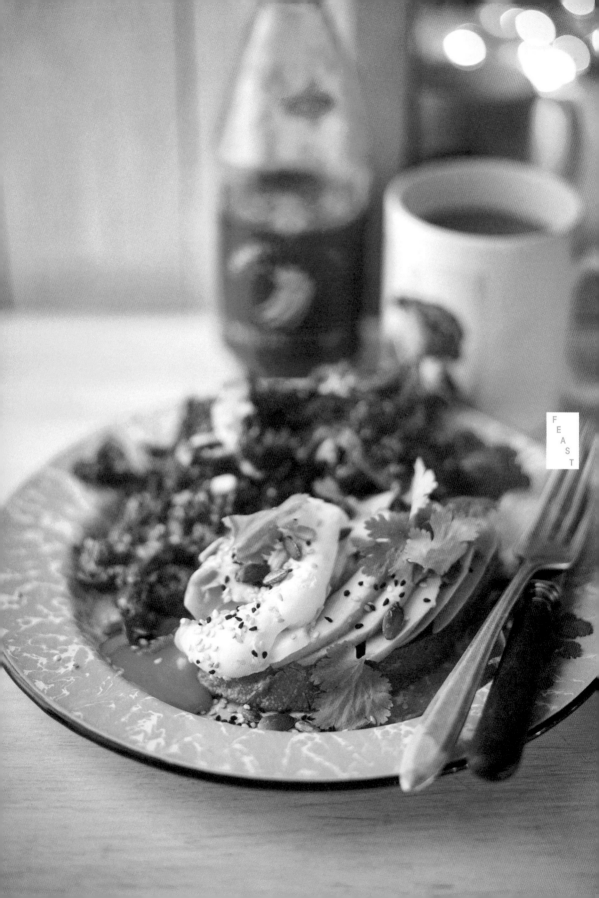

FEAST

Fill your mug with boiling water and leave your tea to brew. Put the toast on.

Heat a glug of olive oil in a large frying pan over a medium heat.

Check that the water in the pan is boiling and using a spoon, start to swirl the water to create a whirlpool. Carefully and with confidence, lower the side of the cup containing the egg as close to the water as possible and slip the egg right into the vortex. Straight away, turn the heat right down so that it's very nearly off. If you're using an electric hob that stays hot long after you've turned it down, move the pan off onto another hob and continue over a very low heat – too vigorous a boil and your egg will burst. The vortex will whip the egg into a neat round. Leave it untouched for 2 minutes, until the white has set and the yolk is still runny.

Meanwhile, put the kale into the preheated frying pan, shake the pan to toss it in the oil and season with salt. Leave to cook for 2 minutes over a medium heat.

The toast should be done by now, so place it on your plate and, using a slotted spoon, carefully lift the egg out of the water and hold it over the pan while all the water runs off the crevices of the egg – you don't want soggy toast. Lay the egg on the toast and arrange the avocado slices alongside.

Tip the kale out of the pan onto the plate.

Sprinkle the whole lot with the seeds and coriander, season everything and drizzle with the Sriracha.

Take the tea bag out of your mug and add the milk (if desired).

Serve. Devour.

Go back to bed.

F
E
A
S
T

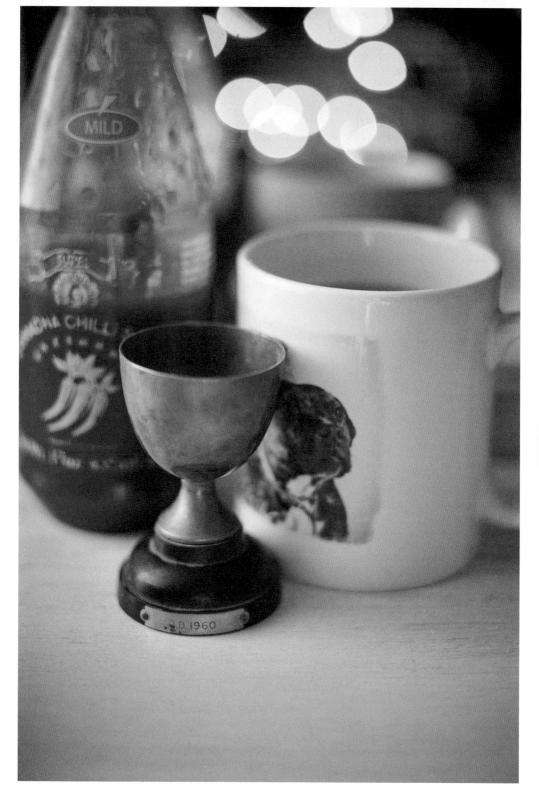

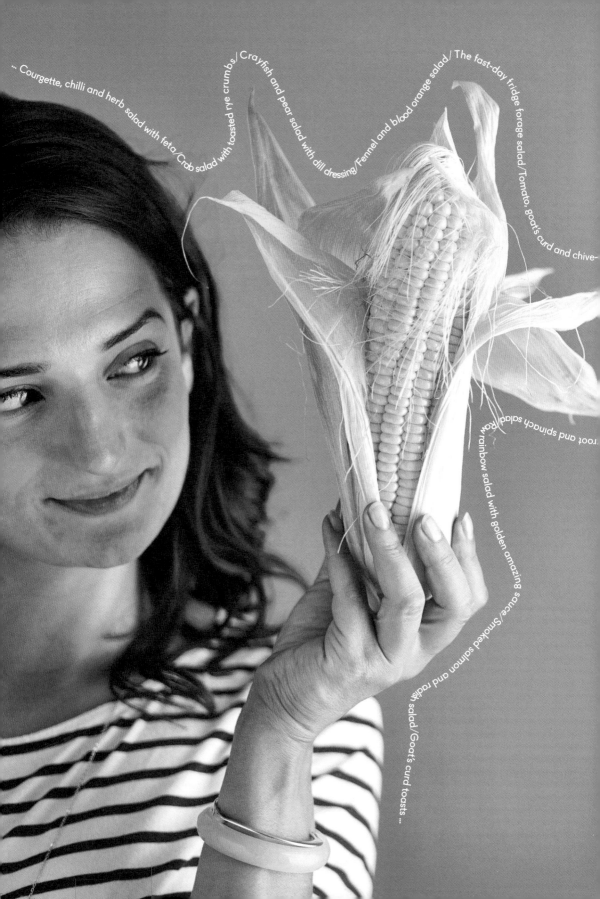

... Courgette, chilli and herb salad with feta / Crab salad with toasted rye crumbs / Crayfish and pear salad with dill dressing / Fennel and blood orange salad / The fast-day fridge forage salad / Tomato, goat's curd and chive-root and spinach salad / Rich rainbow salad with golden amazing sauce / Smoked salmon and radish salad / Goat's curd toasts ...

Weekday Lunches and Salads

Quail eggs, beetroot and spinach salad

A simple, classy salad. Swap the spinach for lettuce or mixed leaves if you like. Add in some asparagus on a fast day for some extra bulk with very few extra calories.

Serves 1
—

3 quail eggs
25g mixed baby leaves
60g cooked beetroot,
    cut into wedges

For the dressing
¼ tsp rapeseed oil
1 tsp red wine vinegar
¼ tsp Dijon mustard
flaked sea salt and freshly
    ground black pepper

To soft-boil the quail eggs, bring a small pan of water to the boil. Gently drop in the eggs and simmer over a medium heat for 40 seconds. Remove with a slotted spoon and immediately plunge into a bowl of ice-cold water. Peel and halve. Set aside.

Whisk the oil, vinegar and mustard in a serving dish. Add the baby leaves and mix to dress.

Add the beetroot and stir to combine.

Top with the eggs, season and serve.

Feast-day variation

On feast days, flake in some hot smoked salmon and slices of cooked new potato.

F
A
S
T

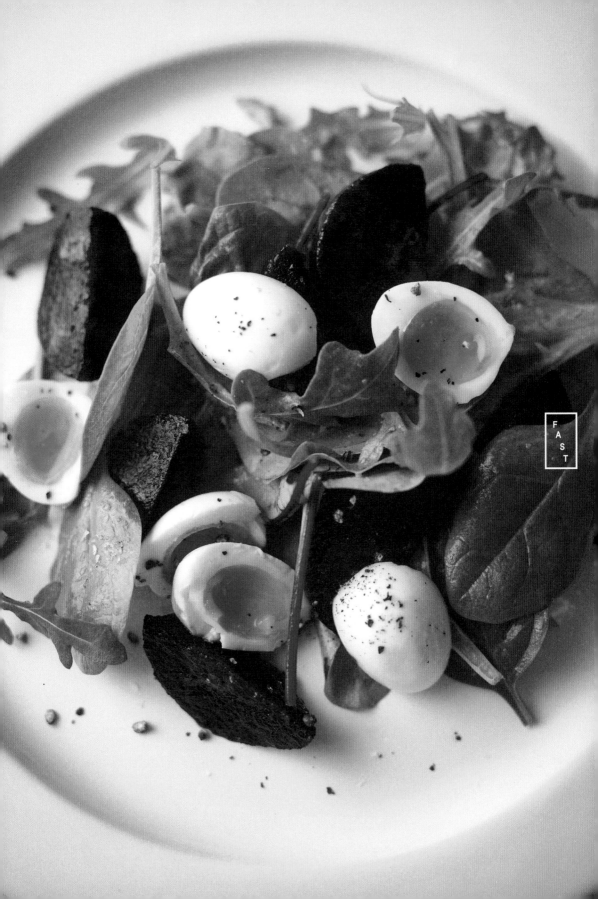

Tomato, goat's curd and chive-flower salad

This is a recreation of the ace lunch I had at one of my favourite restaurants, Silo, in Brighton. They used three different types of tomato, mixed sprouts and a soft, homemade curd made with leftover steamed milk from the coffee bar, which would otherwise be poured away. They are a 'zero waste' restaurant and every time I visit, I learn about something else interesting/creative/inspiring they're doing to avoid throwing anything away. The head chef, Doug, is incredibly generous with his knowledge, and apart from the fact that their food is fantastic, I feel great every time I come away, full of new ideas. This is one to make at that sweet spot near the start of a UK summer, when all the crazy multicoloured heirloom tomatoes start appearing in the greengrocers and the chive flowers are blossoming in the herb pots.

F
A
S
T

Serves 1
—
200g mixture of
    heirloom tomatoes, a
    variety of colours and
    shapes if possible

30g mixed sprouted pulses

25g soft goat's cheese
    or goat's curd

1 tsp Wild Garlic Oil (see
    page 237), or 1 tsp finely
    chopped fresh chives
    mixed with 1 tsp olive oil

chive flowers (optional)

flaked sea salt

Cut the tomatoes at various angles – some in halves, some in slices, some roughly chopped, etc.

Arrange the tomatoes on a plate and scatter the sprouts all over the surface. Season well with salt.

Dot the cheese evenly over the salad and finish with the oil and the chive flowers.

Edamame, pea, miso and ginger salad

This salad would go really well with the Tofu and Kale Gyoza on page 172 to make a light, Japanese-style supper. Adapt the recipe by mixing through some cooked and cooled brown rice (or courgette, either grated or spiralised) and extra dressing and you've got a really nutritious, filling main course. Top with roughly chopped roasted peanuts for added texture, nutrition, contrast and flavour.

Serves 4, as a side

—

110g frozen peas

220g frozen edamame beans

2 x quantity Ginger and Miso Dressing (page 222)

50g carrot, cut into thin matchsticks

20g radish, finely sliced

1 tsp sesame seeds

a few slices of pickled ginger

1 tsp mixed dry seaweed flakes

flaked sea salt

Put the peas and edamame beans in a bowl and pour boiling water over them. Leave to defrost for 5 minutes while you make the rest of the salad.

Drain the peas and beans and put into a serving bowl. Toss with the dressing.

Top with the carrot and radish, then sprinkle with the seeds, pickled ginger and seaweed flakes.

Season with salt and serve.

F
E
A
S
T

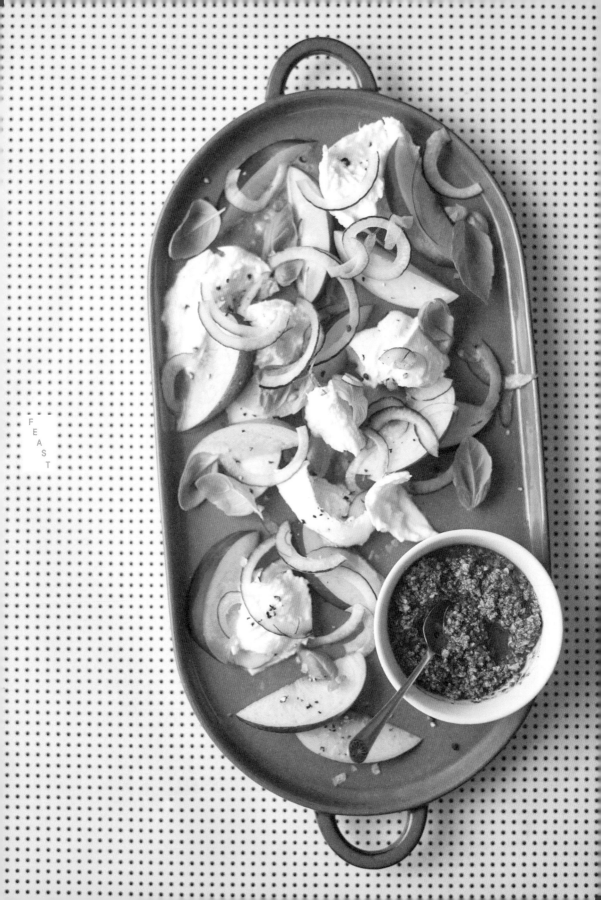

Mozzarella and peach salad with walnut and basil pesto

This salad makes a fabulous summer dinner party starter. You could also serve it as part of a light lunch with a crisp green salad and good bread, or buttery new potatoes.

Serves 4, as a side dish
—

1 x 200g buffalo
   mozzarella

1 ripe peach

10g red onion, very finely
   sliced

a few basil leaves

smoked olive oil, for drizzling

1 x quantity Walnut and
   Basil Pesto (page 236)

smoked salt and freshly
   ground black pepper

Tear the mozzarella into bite-sized pieces and place on a medium-sized platter.

Halve the peach, destone and slice the flesh into wedges. Dot the peach wedges over the plate, sprinkle with the sliced red onion and tear over the basil leaves. Season well.

Finish with a slick of smoked olive oil and dollop the pesto on the side.

F
E
A
S
T

Sweet potato, chickpea and kale salad

Here is a salad that is equally good served warm as soon as you've made it as it is served cold, making it perfect for packed lunches and buffets. The kale keeps its form and doesn't wilt or turn sad.

It's really filling and a complete meal in itself — full of protein, carbohydrates, vitamins and minerals. If you want to add something else to it, flaked smoked mackerel works very well.

Serves 6

—

500g sweet potato

1 red onion

2 tbsp olive oil

150g short-grain brown rice

5 tbsp Pear Café Dressing (see page 227)

100g kale, stems removed and leaves roughly torn into bite-sized pieces

30g pumpkin seeds

1 x 400g tin chickpeas, drained and rinsed

30g raw beetroot, grated

1 small handful of coriander, leaves picked

1 small handful of flat-leaf parsley, leaves picked

flaked sea salt and freshly ground black pepper

Preheat the oven to 200°C/400°F/Gas mark 6.

Peel both the sweet potato and the onion and cut them into 1–2cm cubes.

Put in a roasting tray lined with baking parchment and drizzle with the olive oil. Holding opposite corners of the baking parchment, bring them together and toss the vegetables in the oil. Season with salt and pepper. Roast in the oven for 30 minutes, until the sweet potato is charred.

Meanwhile, weigh the rice in a measuring jug and check where it comes up to under ml. Rinse well in cold water and drain. Tip into a saucepan and add three times the volume of boiling water from the kettle. Stir once and bring up to the boil over high heat. Stir once more and cover with a lid. Turn the heat right down to minimum and simmer for 25 minutes, or until the rice is tender to bite.

While the rice and the vegetables are cooking, get the rest of the salad ready.

Pour the dressing into a large serving bowl and add the ripped-up kale. Using your hands, rub the dressing into the kale for a full minute. This will soften the kale while allowing it to keep all its raw goodness.

Add most of the pumpkin seeds, the chickpeas and the beetroot. Season well and toss. Drain the rice well and add to the bowl. Take the sweet potato and red onion out of the oven and mix everything up really well. Sprinkle the remaining pumpkin seeds and the herbs over the top. Serve.

Mexican avocado chopped salad

You can use this creamy dressing on loads of things. I particularly like it in a chopped salad like this. There's so much going on here – textures, flavours, colours – and it's packed full of nutrients.

Thanks to the beans, this really is a substantial salad and the recipe makes one huge portion. Use the rest of the corn to make the Blueberry, Avocado and Corn Salad (page 77) and take it to work as a packed lunch, or make a small batch of the Sweetcorn, Chipotle and Buckwheat Fritters on page 43.

Serves 1

---

2 large handfuls Romaine, cos or little gem lettuce, cut into 2.5cm wide ribbons

4 cherry tomatoes, quartered

¼ ripe avocado, quartered

¼ red or orange pepper, deseeded and diced

2 tbsp sweetcorn kernels

2 tbsp black beans

½ red onion, finely diced

For the dressing (makes enough for 4 portions)

¾ ripe avocado, destoned

2 garlic cloves

2 tbsp apple cider vinegar

60ml olive oil

2 tbsp toasted pumpkin seeds

1 tsp cumin

juice of 2 limes

1 tsp chipotle chilli flakes, or ¼ tsp fresh red chilli, very finely chopped

handful of chopped fresh coriander (including stalks)

2 generous pinches of flaked sea salt

To serve

1 tbsp sunflower seeds, toasted

2 lime wedges

flaked sea salt and freshly ground black pepper

First, make the dressing by simply throwing the ingredients into a blender and blitzing until smooth. Add a splash or two of water until it's as smooth as you want it. The dressing keeps well in the fridge in a well-sealed jar for up to 3 days if you want to make this in advance.

Lay the lettuce on a serving bowl and toss the remaining ingredients together. Top the lettuce with the chopped vegetables, add the toppings and serve with the dressing on the side.

Variation

The salad is also incredible served with a small handful of tortilla chips (see page 77). The leftover salad dressing can be used as a dip for the chips. Do it.

Alternatively, add a sprinkling of cheese (feta, Cheddar or Parmesan shavings all work well). The Cajun Prawns on page 160 would make a great addition, too.

FEAST

Raw rainbow salad
with golden amazing sauce

This is gluten-free and vegan (if those things matter to you). It's enormous and delicious (those things matter to everyone), and it's less than 100 calories. Add some king prawns to the top for a more substantial – but still very low-calorie – fast-day meal, or mix some Spicy Roasted Chickpeas (page 201) through the salad for even more crunch on feast days.

I made the salad in the winter, but you can make it all year round – just use what you can find and recalculate the calories carefully. NB: High water-content veg will always be the lowest in calories. Crunchy things like red pepper, chicory and carrot would all work really well in this salad. Get as many colours in there as possible. Eat the rainbow, dudes!

Serves 1

———

50g fennel

30g raw beetroot (any colour, but golden or stripy looks best in this)

40g red cabbage

50g broccoli

15g celery, plus leaves if possible

15g apple, finely sliced

25g mixed sprouts

10g Golden Amazing Sauce (see page 220)

1 tbsp sherry vinegar

2g furikake (Japanese rice seasoning)

flaked sea salt and freshly ground black pepper

Slice the fennel, beetroot and cabbage very finely, using a mandoline if you have one, or a very sharp knife. Place in a bowl.

Chop the broccoli into very fine florets, running your knife over the pile in both directions until you have pieces just slightly bigger than broccoli 'rice'. Add this to the bowl with the apple and sprouts. Season well and toss all together.

Transfer to your serving bowl and drizzle with the Golden Amazing Sauce and the sherry vinegar.

Sprinkle over the furikake and serve.

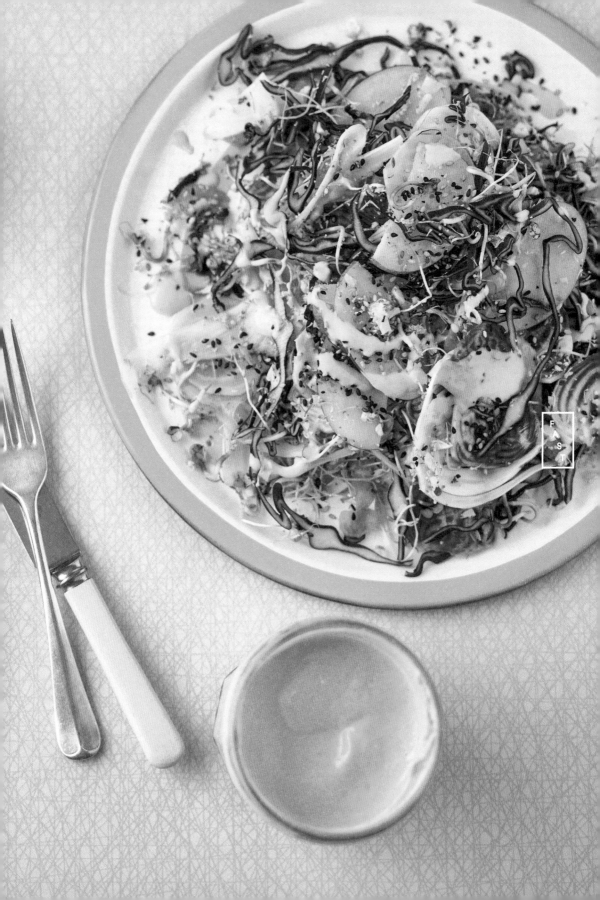

Prawn, mango and jalapeño salad

101 kcal per portion

Serves 1

- 60g cooked prawns (king prawns if possible)
- 30g mango, cut into 1cm dice
- 10g pickled jalapeños from a jar, very finely chopped
- 20g baby spinach
- 15g rocket
- 7g China rose radish sprouts (or use 25g alfalfa)
- 1 tsp lemon juice
- flaked sea salt and freshly ground black pepper
- ¼ tsp extra-virgin olive oil

F A S T

Combine all ingredients except the extra-virgin olive oil in a large bowl.

Toss well and taste for seasoning, then drizzle with the oil.

If you are making this in advance, for a packed lunch, remove from the fridge about half an hour before eating to give it a chance to come to room temperature. It'll taste much better if it's not fridge-cold.

Raw winter veg salad

86 kcal
per portion

Serves 1

———

50g fennel

50g blood orange

40g chicory

40g raw beetroot
(golden or regular)

8g rocket

1 tsp extra-virgin olive oil

1 tsp sherry vinegar

flaked sea salt and freshly
ground black pepper

Rinse the fennel well. Cut it in half from top to bottom. Use a mandoline or a very sharp knife to slice very thinly. Put 50g in a large bowl. Wrap the rest in cling film and stick it in the fridge.

Cut the top and bottom off the orange and stand it up on the board. Using a sharp knife, cut off the skin and pith, running your knife in small sawing movements from top to bottom, working your way around the fruit. Cut the orange into slices and weigh out 50g. Add to the bowl. Wrap the rest in cling film and stick it in the fridge.

Cut the base off the chicory and separate the leaves. Wash and spin dry. Weigh out 40g. Add to the bowl. Wrap the rest in cling film and stick it in the fridge.

Peel the raw beetroot. Use a mandoline or a very sharp knife to slice very thinly. Put 40g in a large bowl. Wrap the rest and stick it in the fridge.

Add the rocket to the bowl and season well. Toss it all together and drizzle with the oil and vinegar.

Refrigerate until you're ready to eat, but try to take the salad out of the fridge about half an hour before to allow the salad to come to room temperature. It'll taste much better if it's not fridge-cold.

F
A
S
T

Crayfish and pear salad with dill dressing

172 kcal per portion

How did I end up with so many hot Scandi mates? They're all mega-clever and talented, too. I don't know, but I'm not complaining. I made this while daydreaming of hot Swedish summers, jumping in the lake at Marielund with my best mate, Cissy.

Whole crayfish are delicious, but a right pain in the neck to eat. Buy a tub of ready-to-eat (peeled and cooked) crayfish tails and save yourself about three days' worth of work.

This makes a huge salad — easily enough to serve two as a lunch or a starter. If you're on a fast day, it makes a generous dinner for one. I'd serve it with buttered rye bread or crispbreads if I made it on a feast day. Or try new potatoes boiled with dill, dressed with butter and tossed through the salad to make a much more filling dish.

Serves 1

60g piece of cucumber
20g pear
¼ tsp lemon juice
25g rocket
125g crayfish tails
60g little gem or cos lettuce, rinsed, dried well and leaves separated
flaked sea salt and freshly ground black pepper

FAST

For the dressing

¼ tsp Dijon mustard

¼ tsp wholegrain mustard

¼ tsp runny honey

1 tsp white wine vinegar

1 tsp extra-virgin olive oil

a few sprigs of dill,
    finely chopped

In a small bowl, combine the mustards, honey, vinegar and olive oil. Whisk well. Thin with a little water if the dressing is too thick to drizzle.

Add half the finely chopped dill and whisk.

Use a vegetable peeler to create long ribbons of cucumber (or finely slice with your mandoline) and place them in a bowl.

Cut the pear into wafer-thin slices and add them to the bowl, too. Sprinkle over the lemon juice to stop the pear discolouring. Add the rocket and the crayfish. Season well and toss it all together. Lay the lettuce out on your serving plate and top with the contents of the bowl. Drizzle with the dressing and add the remaining dill all over the top. Serve.

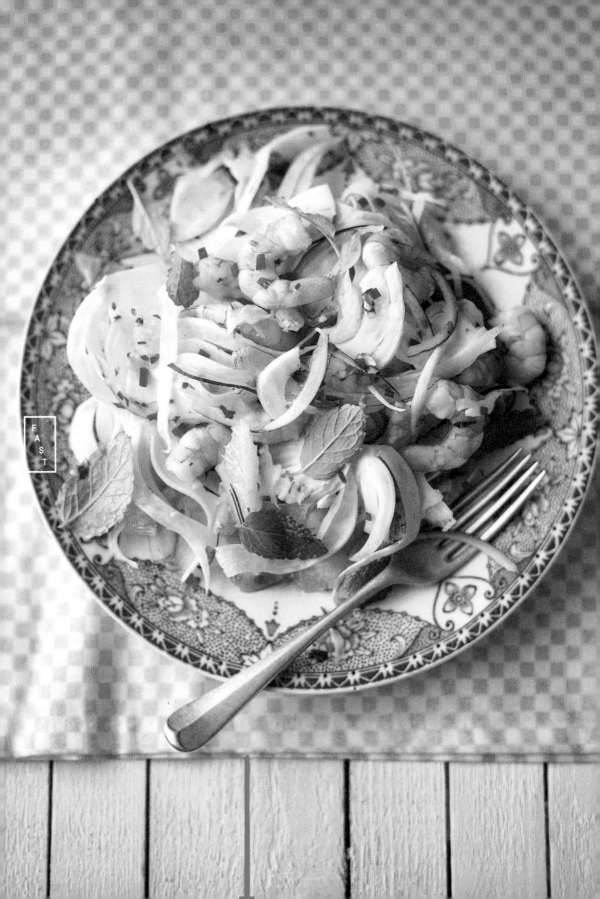

King prawn, fennel, pink grapefruit and mint salad

177 kcal
per portion

Packets of pre-marinated prawns are a great fast-day staple. Look carefully at the ingredients list and if there's anything in the list you couldn't buy yourself off the shop shelves, put it back. That means spices, herbs, lemon, garlic, etc. are all cool; E numbers are not.

Serves 1

—

80g fennel

130g ready-cooked marinated king prawns

50g pink grapefruit, segmented

10g red onion, very thinly sliced

1g finely chopped mint

1g finely diced red chilli

flaked sea salt and freshly ground black pepper

Slice the fennel very finely, using a mandoline or a very sharp knife. Put in a bowl with the remaining ingredients and mix well, squeezing the grapefruit membrane over the salad.

Season well and serve.

F
A
S
T

107 kcal
per portion

Crab salad with toasted rye crumbs

White crab meat is hugely less calorific than the brown meat. You can buy a tub of white meat only in the supermarket and lots of fishmongers sell it, too. The watercress and radish make this quite a sharp combo, and I love the contrast of the toasted rye breadcrumbs against the soft crab meat. If you want to take this in to work, make the salad and keep the breadcrumbs separate, wrapped in a little cling-film pouch. Sprinkle them on when you're ready to eat. You can swap the rye crumbs for standard breadcrumbs — just make sure you recalculate the calories.

Serves 1

—

1 slice rye bread

20g fennel

1 tsp lemon juice

10g spring onion, finely sliced

15g radish, finely sliced

5g red chilli, finely sliced

100g cooked white crab meat

1 tbsp roughly chopped flat-leaf parsley

3g mint, whole leaves picked

25g watercress

flaked sea salt and freshly ground black pepper

F
A
S
T

To make the rye crumbs, blitz the bread in a food processor until you have fine crumbs.

Slice the fennel very finely, using a mandoline or a very sharp knife. Put into a mixing bowl and squeeze over the lemon juice.

Finely slice the spring onion, radish and chilli and add to the bowl.

Flake in the crab meat and add the herbs.

Carefully fold everything together (you don't want to mush up the crab) and add the watercress. Season well.

Toast the breadcrumbs in a dry pan until golden brown and crunchy.

Transfer the salad to a serving dish and top with the toasted breadcrumbs.

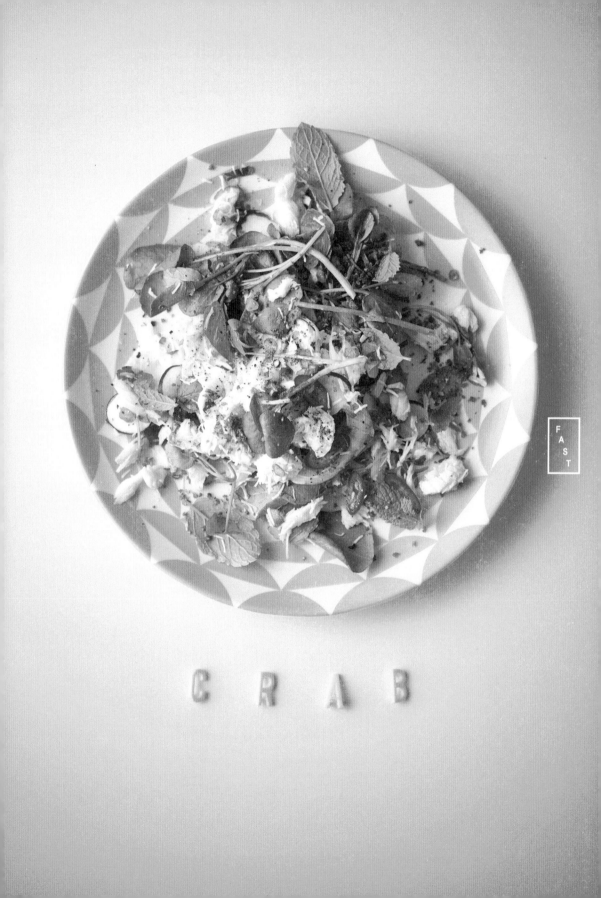

FAST

CRAB

91 kcal
per portion

Smoked salmon and radish salad

A few delicate, peppery, crunchy garnishes on top of the best-quality smoked salmon you can afford, this dish is as pretty as a picture and every mouthful really packs a punch. It's also one of the few fast-day recipes that I'd do in exactly the same way if I was serving it on a feast day.

Serves 1
—

60g smoked salmon

20g radish

3g spring onion,
    sliced on the diagonal

10g China rose radish
    sprouts

⅛ tsp poppy seeds

1 tsp lemon juice

freshly ground black pepper

1g fennel fronds

Lay the salmon out on a serving plate, creating a neat circle.

Slice the radish very thinly, using a very sharp knife or a mandoline.

Lay the radish slices evenly over the surface of the salmon. Sprinkle over the spring onion.

Scatter the sprouts and the poppy seeds over the top and sprinkle with the lemon juice.

Season well with black pepper and finish with the delicate fennel fronds.

F
A
S
T

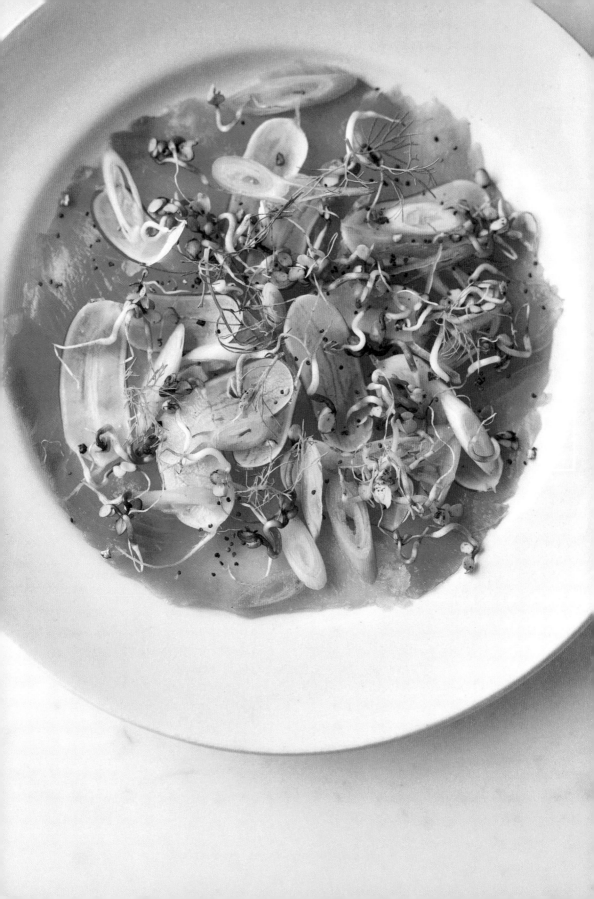

100-calorie packed lunch boxes

~~~~~

I understand that (especially) when you first start the 5:2 and you're finding your feet, there's quite a bit to learn. However, I beg you not to fall into just eating ready meals and convenience foods. The whole idea of cooking properly on fast days is that you're educating yourself and learning how to make better, healthier choices on feast days. Understanding what goes into your food is essential.

Getting organised really helps. Before starting the 5:2, I'd suggest really trying to clear out your fridge. Make space for what's going to be your new way of eating.

Go shopping. Invest in (or dig out) some Tupperware and zip-lock bags. Come home and prepare all the fresh stuff. This is what we do at my café and it's definitely the way to go. If all your veg is washed, trimmed and prepared, you can make healthy meals really quickly and it takes up less room in the fridge. I'd suggest, for example, going shopping at the weekend, doing your meal prep on Sunday night and doing your fast day on the Monday. Remember – you are going to measure and weigh everything really carefully for your fast-day meals, but on your feast days you don't need to calculate anything at all. The clever thing is,

though, if your fridge is full of lovely fresh stuff, you'll eat well anyway. As you make the 100-kcal boxes, put any leftover bits into a Tupperware or in a zip-lock bag. Look at my Fast-day Fridge Forage Salad guide on page 82 for guidance on what to do with all the bits and pieces you're left with. Nothing will get wasted, trust me.

These boxes have been carefully calculated to equal exactly 100 kcal each. Women are allowed 500 kcal on a fast day and men are allowed 600 kcal. The best way to do it would be to make four boxes (so 400 kcal in total), take a couple to work with you and leave a couple at home. If you only feel like eating one during the day, bring the second one home for later. Until you start the 5:2, it's hard to know what will work best for you with regards to how you lay out your day. I generally save most of my calories for the evening, but I know others who choose to 'front load' and prefer to eat earlier. If you have four boxes prepared, you've still got 100 kcal (or 200 kcal, bros) left for drinks, snacks, etc. Just don't screw it all up. Weigh and measure everything out carefully. It's just for today, for tomorrow we feast!

You can make any of the boxes up to 24 hours before you want to eat them. Any longer and they'll go a bit sad.

Blueberry, avocado and corn salad

100 kcal
per portion

This is a fantastically easy side salad. Add a little feta (10g for 28 kcal) or the Cajun Prawns from page 160 to make this into a main course salad.

Makes 4 portions

165g tinned sweetcorn, drained

100g blueberries

100g cucumber, diced

45g red onion, finely diced

10g roughly chopped coriander

20g pickled jalapeños, roughly chopped

30g avocado, finely diced

1 tbsp lime juice

1 tbsp olive oil

¼ tsp ground cumin

¼ tsp salt

a few turns of black pepper

Simply tip all the ingredients into a bowl and fold together carefully, then eat immediately or place in an airtight container and refrigerate until needed.

a #100calorielunchbox recipe

F
A
S
T

Courgette, chilli and herb salad with feta

100 kcal
per portion

Makes 1 portion

175g mixed yellow and green courgettes

juice of ½ lemon

¼ tsp extra-virgin olive oil

¼ tsp red chilli, finely diced

a few mint leaves (mostly roughly chopped, a few small leaves left whole), coriander and basil leaves

15g feta

flaked sea salt and freshly ground black pepper

Grate the courgettes into a serving bowl.

Squeeze the lemon juice over the courgettes and season well.

Drizzle with the oil, scatter over the chilli and chopped mint and stir to combine.

Add the whole mint leaves and the remaining herbs.

Crumble the feta over the top, and serve.

a #100calorielunchbox recipe

Fennel and blood orange salad

In late January and early February, blood oranges will appear in the grocers. Grab them while you can – their fantastic colour brings a much-needed shot of brightness in the cold, grey months and they're not around for long. I tend to find that the ones that show the most red on their skin seem to be the 'bloodiest' inside, but maybe I've just been lucky.

Serves 1

—

100g fennel

a pinch of flaked sea salt

50g blood orange segments

15g pomegranate seeds

3g pistachios, dry toasted
    in a frying pan, then
    roughly chopped.

2.5ml extra-virgin olive oil

freshly ground black pepper

a few small mint leaves

Slice the fennel very thinly, using a mandoline or a very sharp knife. Sprinkle with salt.

Add the orange segments, pomegranate seeds and nuts.

Toss gently and transfer to a small serving plate.

Drizzle with the olive oil, season, then add the mint.

a #100calorielunchbox recipe

F
A
S
T

Smoked trout and cauliflower rice salad

87 kcal
per portion

If you've opened a packet of smoked trout, the remainder will be fine
to freeze. Just seal it carefully in a zip-lock bag and defrost it in the fridge.

Serves 1
—

100g cauliflower

4g coriander, finely
chopped

1g spring onion

40g smoked trout

¼ lemon, for squeezing

flaked sea salt and freshly
ground black pepper

First, make the cauliflower rice, following the instructions
on page 16.

Once done, tip the cauliflower rice into a bowl and let
it cool, then fold through the coriander and spring onion
and flake in the trout. Fold gently so it doesn't end up
a big mushed-up mess. Taste for seasoning. Bag up the
remaining raw cauliflower rice into portions and label
and freeze them.

Wipe out the pan and put it back on the heat. When it's
hot, put the lemon in, cut side down, and hold it in place,
keeping it totally still. You want to hold it down over the
heat until it starts to blacken and caramelise. (This way
you get a nice smoky flavour when you squeeze it over
the salad.) Once it's done, fill your box with the cauliflower
and trout mixture and tuck the lemon in the corner.

Refrigerate until you're ready to eat, but try to take the
salad out of the fridge about half an hour before to allow
it to come to room temperature. It'll taste much better
if it's not fridge-cold. Squeeze the lemon over and eat.

F
A
S
T

a #100calorielunchbox recipe

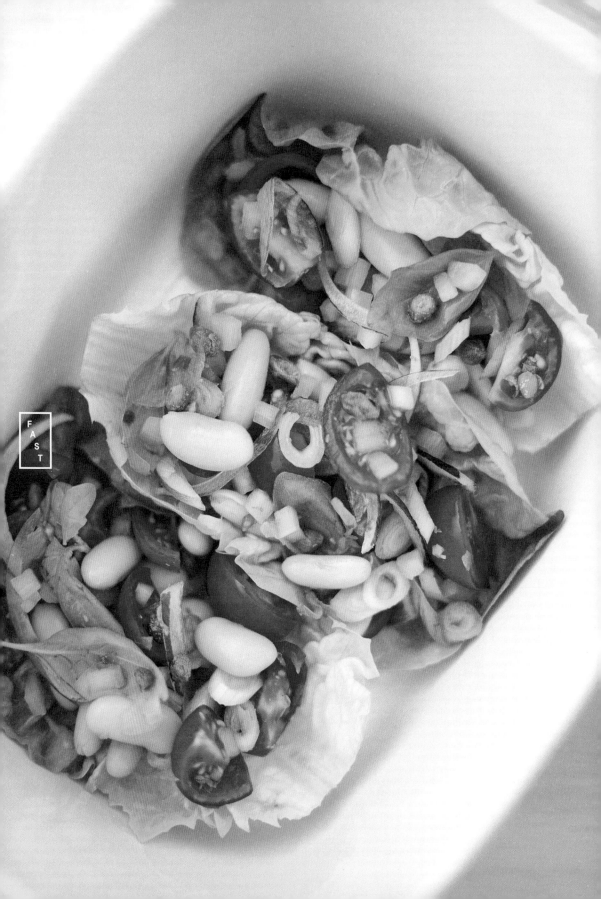

FAST

Cannellini bean salad in little gem cups

93 kcal per portion

Serves 2
—

1 x 400g tin cannellini beans, drained and well rinsed

50g spring onion, sliced

1 tbsp lemon juice

130g cherry tomatoes, quartered

15g mini capers, or roughly chopped regular capers

10g basil leaves

15g red onion, very finely sliced

40g celery, very finely diced

flaked sea salt and freshly ground black pepper

6 little gem lettuce leaves (total 60g)

Combine all the ingredients apart from the lettuce in a bowl.

Lay three lettuce leaves in each box and distribute the bean salad evenly.

a #100calorielunchbox recipe

F
A
S
T

The fast-day fridge forage salad

This isn't a recipe. It's a guide. When I posted a picture of this salad on Instagram, people went nuts over it.

I was making dinner for me and my then-housemate, Bev. We'd pooled our fridge leftovers and I prepped everything, laid it all out and we made our own salads. She's not on the 5:2, so filled her bowl with joyous abandon. I, on the other hand, had to take a bit longer doing it carefully, but it wasn't hard. You just need to be organised.

I can't give you a calorie count for this one. It entirely depends on what you have in your fridge and what you put in your version. What I can do is tell you which foods make good ingredients for a fast-day salad and give you some tips and ideas on how to prepare them.

Use whatever you have on hand to make this salad — that's the fun and foraging part of it. Here are some ideas on how to put them together.

Serves 2, plus leftovers

—

250g cauliflower

1 small bunch of coriander

2 eggs

70g little gem lettuce

100g asparagus

25g rocket

60g courgette

40g kale

120g smoked trout

25g red cabbage

1 spring onion

60g fennel

10g red onion

15g China rose radish sprouts

20g mixed bean sprouts

40g Greek yoghurt

1 tsp extra-virgin olive oil

1 tsp balsamic vinegar

1 tbsp furikake (Japanese rice seasoning)

flaked sea salt and freshly ground black pepper

First, empty your fridge and decide what you're going to use. Write down everything. Put back the stuff you're not going to use. Use a calorie-counting app like MyFitnessPal to look everything up. This is the boring but very important bit. When you need to input weights, at this point you can guess roughly what you'll be using for now. Now, prepare everything as directed, doing the hot stuff last. Lay it all out on the table or counter. Get a bowl and put it on the scales. Start assembling your salad, working down the list you've created in the app and adjusting the weights until they're all in there accurately. For example, I guessed I'd be using about 100g of trout, but when I started adding it to the bowl 45g looked plenty, so I adjusted the entry and it dropped down from 150 kcal to 68 kcal.

How you arrange the salad is up to you, but I like to keep each main ingredient in its own little section of the bowl and then finish it off with the garnishes and seasonings.

And that's it. Eat the salad.

Once you've made your salad, gather up any prepared leftover pieces into a Tupperware box and stick it in the fridge. You've got the basis of tomorrow's packed lunch ready to go. I took the tub to work the next day and made a big salad, tipping all the delicious extras on top.

Tips & ingredient ideas

You want to get as many different textures and flavours into the salad as possible, so use a knife, a mandoline, a grater, a peeler – even your hands – to cut up the ingredients in as many ways as you can.

High water-content veg are the lowest in calories. Things like lettuce, fennel, courgette ribbons, asparagus, etc., are ridiculously low. Use these to compose the main bulk of your salad.

Get some protein in there. Boiled eggs, flaked smoked trout and chickpeas are all good.

Some warm/hot elements are a nice touch. I make cauliflower rice (with added coriander, see 16, and some stir-fried kale.

Dressings. Greek yoghurt, extra-virgin olive oil, balsamic vinegar and furikake (Japanese rice seasoning) are all great ideas for dressings.

Think about garnishes. I'm a big fan of a good garnish, especially on fast days. They add flavour, texture and visual interest. Taking time to really present your food as well as possible makes fast days so much more satisfying.

F
A
S
T

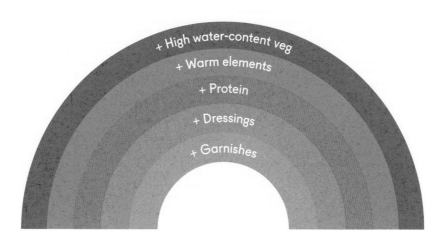

Goat's curd toasts

Believe it or not, these pretty little toasts started life as the result of a fridge forage. I was about to go away and had all sorts of nice bits and pieces I wanted to use up before I left. Some of it was stuff I'd picked in the park from the brilliant Edible Bristol scheme, in which flowerbeds in public spaces are planted with vegetables, herbs and edible flowers that people are welcome to help themselves to. I picked the borage flowers and the fennel tops and brought them home in my hand, being careful not to crush them. I picked the herbs from my rooftop herb boxes and dug the bread out of the freezer. The goat's curd was the end of a pot (the tartness of the curd contrasts so well with the sweet peach), but a soft goat's cheese or cream cheese would work well, too.

Use toast, peach and cheese as the base, but feel free to switch the other ingredients, with the exception of the smoked salt and spring onion, which I see as an essential as they tone down the sweetness. Other soft herbs would work, too. The edible flowers are an optional addition, but the chive flowers are more than just decorative — they have a wonderful flavour that falls somewhere between spring onion, chive and shallot. If you can't get them, use a bit of one (or all) of these to replace them.

This makes a very classy, light, summery lunch with a green or tomato salad. Alternatively, use bite-sized pieces of toast to make beautiful canapés.

Serves 2 as a light lunch, or makes 24 canapés

---

4 slices of sourdough bread

4 tbsp goat's curd

¼ peach, destoned and thinly sliced

a few sprigs of basil

a few chive flowers

a few borage flowers

a few mint leaves

a small sprig of fennel tops

1 spring onion, finely sliced

smoked salt and freshly ground black pepper

Toast the bread, spread each slice with the goat's curd and lay the peach slices on top.

Scatter with the remaining ingredients and season to taste.

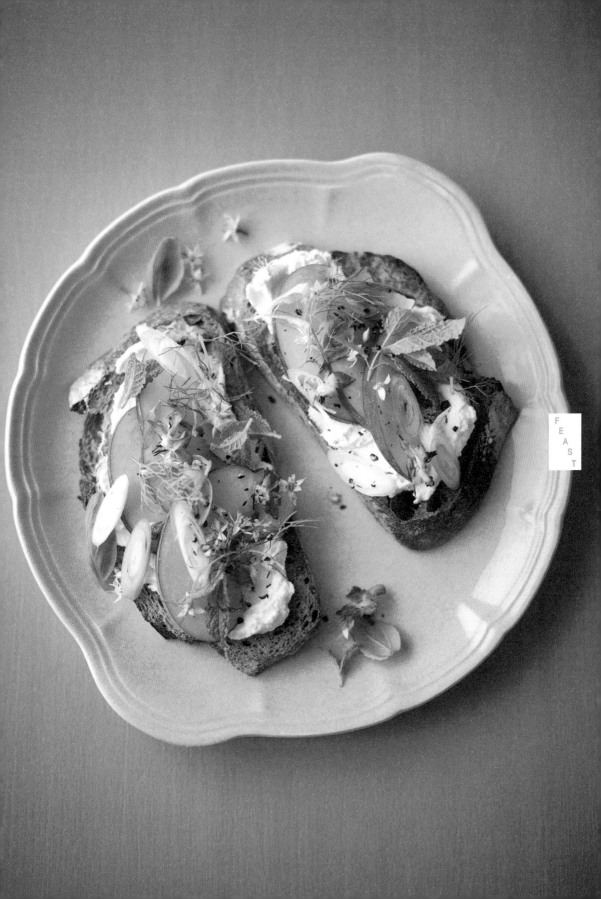

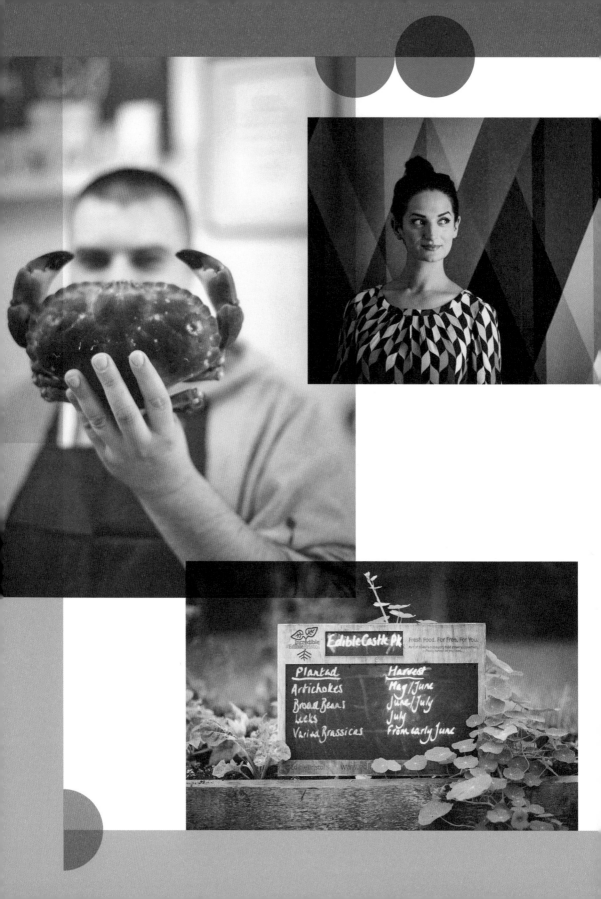

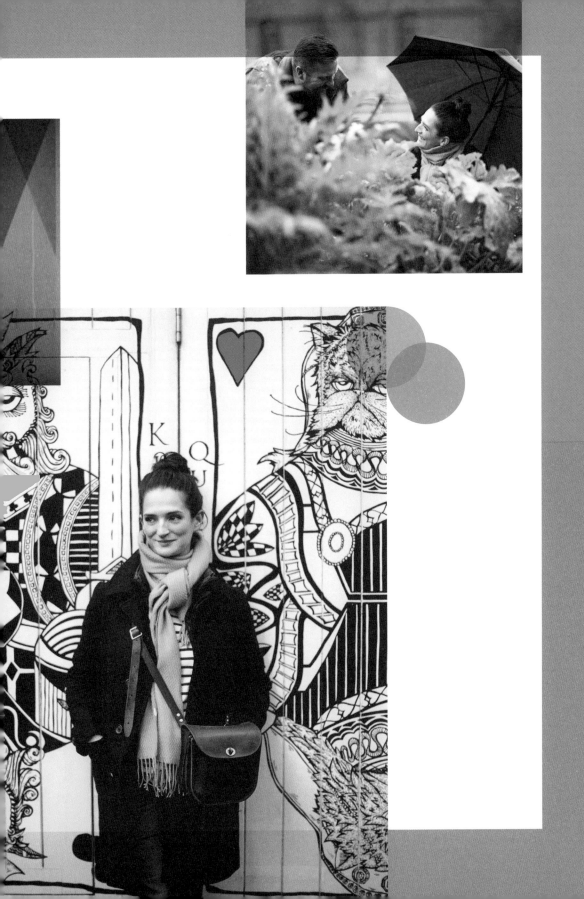

Pea, potato, feta and seed salad

This salad is a regular feature on the café's outside catering menus. It's always popular, easy to make and happy at any temperature.

I developed the technique for crushing the peas so that they would cling to the spuds rather than roll through the gaps and fall to the bottom of the bowl. Crushing the peas also helps to get their flavour out – or, as long-time café babe Sophie very innocently explained to then-new-girl Steph, it helps to 'release the pea-ness'. It's true, it does.

Serves 4, as a side dish

500g new potatoes, scrubbed
200g frozen peas
2 tbsp olive oil
100g feta
2 tbsp Pear Café Seed Blend (see page 227)
a few mint leaves
1 tsp finely chopped red chilli
flaked sea salt and freshly ground black pepper

Slice the potatoes in half, and any large ones into quarters.

Place in a pan with just enough water to cover. Add a pinch of salt. Bring to the boil over a high heat, reduce to a medium-low heat and cook, covered, for 8–12 minutes or until the potatoes are tender.

Cook the peas in a pan of boiling water, according to the packet instructions. Immediately drain in a sieve and run under cold water – this will stop them cooking and preserve their greenness.

Put the cooked peas in a serving bowl and add 1 tablespoon olive oil. Using a potato masher, crush the peas lightly, leaving some whole. Season well with plenty of sea salt and black pepper. Mix well.

Add the potatoes and stir to combine.

Crumble over half of the feta and carefully fold in. Add the remaining feta over the top, sprinkle with the seeds and garnish with the mint leaves, chopped chilli, remaining olive oil and a little extra salt.

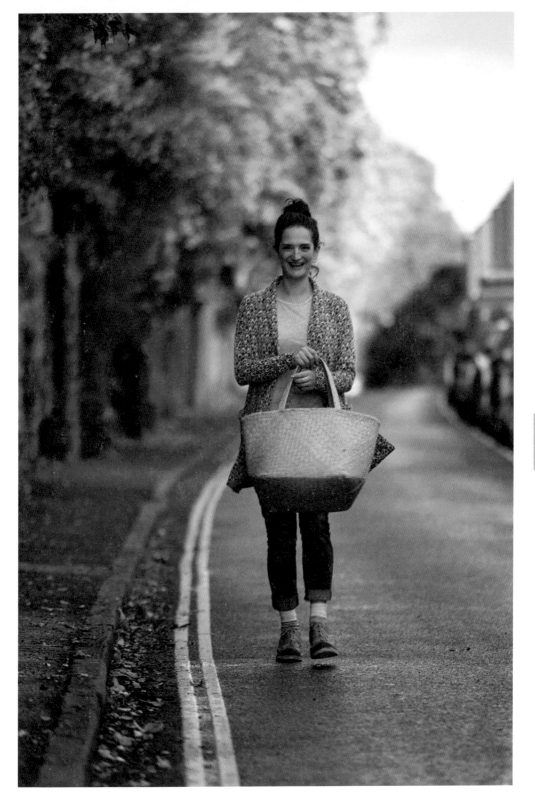

Pear Café frittata

We make frittata every day at the Pear Café and it always sells out. There are so many things that make frittata great. It's happy left out of the fridge for a couple of hours, so it's perfect for picnics or packed lunches. It's cheap and easy to make. You can add almost anything – it's a great way to use up leftovers, and you can play around with the basic recipe to your own tastes. I've included four variations here, but look on Instagram under pearcafefrittata for loads more inspiration.

Base mixture

Serves 8
—

12 medium new potatoes
1 tbsp unsalted butter
1 tbsp olive oil, plus extra
6 eggs
250g mature Cheddar, grated
flaked sea salt and freshly ground black pepper

Fill a pan with water and add the potatoes. Bring to the boil and cook for 15 minutes over a medium heat until tender. Drain and allow to cool. Slice into thick discs.

Heat the butter and oil in a 25cm non-stick frying pan. Fry the potatoes for 10–15 minutes, until golden brown on both sides. Allow to cool.

Break the eggs into a large jug and whisk well. Add 3 tablespoons water to the eggs, along with a large pinch of salt and a good few turns of black pepper. Whisk well and stir in the cheese.

Add the fried potatoes to the jug and stir well.

The frittata base mixture is finished. Continue, following the instructions overleaf for any of the variations.

To cook the frittata, preheat the grill and heat a splash of olive oil in the frying pan used to fry your potatoes. When hot, pour in the egg mixture. Using a heatproof rubber spatula, gently drag the edges towards the centre, tipping the pan and letting the liquid eggs flow into the gap you have created. This helps the whole thing set, rather than just the bottom of the frittata. Continue doing this for 5 minutes, until almost set and the top is still liquid.

Place the pan under the grill (making sure the handle is not under the grill if it is plastic) and grill until golden. Remove and set aside to cool in the pan for 5 minutes.

Slide the frittata out gently onto a chopping board and set aside for 5 more minutes. To serve, slice into eight pieces. This is very good warm or cold.

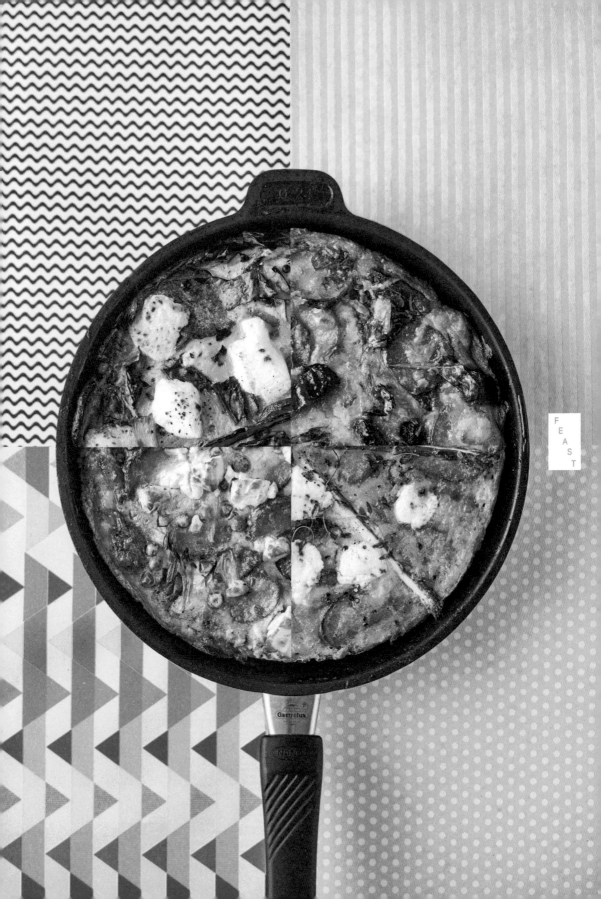

FEAST

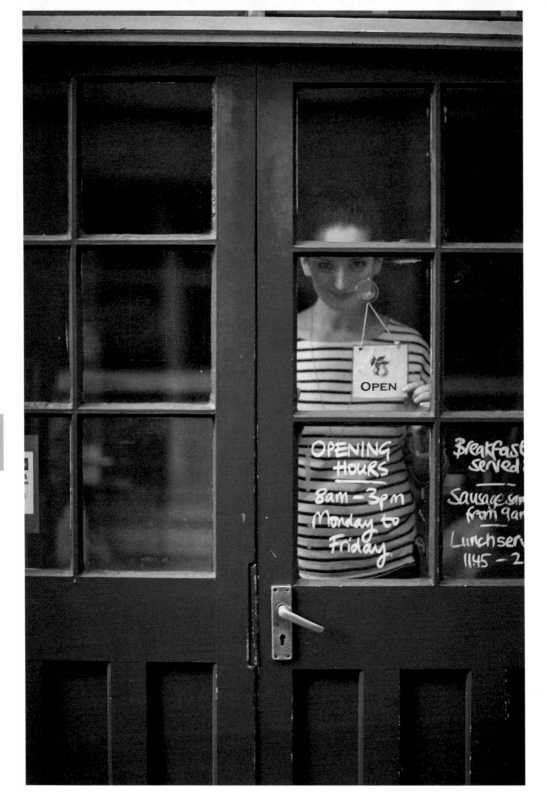

Beetroot, spinach and halloumi

2 cooked beetroot, cubed
1 large handful of baby
spinach
125g halloumi, grated
1 tbsp olive oil

Follow the basic recipe on page 90, adding the cooked beetroot cubes, spinach and two-thirds of the halloumi to the whisked eggs, and stir well. Sprinkle the surface of the fritatta with the remaining halloumi before grilling.

Pea, feta and spring onion

1 cup cooked peas
3 spring onions, finely sliced
⅓ pack feta, crumbled

Follow the basic recipe on page 90, stirring the peas and spring onions into the egg mixture. Sprinkle the surface of the frittata with feta before grilling.

Asparagus and goat's cheese

a few springs of fresh thyme,
leaves picked
4 asparagus spears, cut
lengthways and rubbed
with a little olive oil
50g soft goat's cheese

Follow the basic recipe on page 90, stirring the thyme into the egg mixture. Lay the asparagus and small chunks of goat's cheese evenly across the surface of the frittata before grilling.

F
E
A
S
T

Rainbow chard, courgette and goat's cheese

1 bunch of rainbow chard,
rinsed and drained well
knob of unsalted butter,
for frying
1 courgette, grated
100g soft goat's cheese

Cut the stalks off the chard and cut them into 10cm lengths, cutting the wider stalks in half lengthways, too. Pile the chard leaves on top of each other and roll them up. Cut into 2cm ribbons and set aside.

Melt the butter in the frying pan you'll use for the frittata and add the stalks. Fry for 5 minutes, over a medium heat, until softened. Remove and allow to cool briefly.

Follow the basic recipe on page 90, stirring the grated courgette, chard stalks and leaves into the egg mixture. Tear small chunks of goat's cheese evenly over the surface of the frittata before grilling.

Grandma's egg and onion

There's a recording studio round the corner from the café and when musicians are recording there John and Ali, who run it, often bring them to the café for lunch. We've met loads of great people from all over the world. One of our all-time favourites was American artist Trevor Powers (aka Youth Lagoon). For almost two months, he came in nearly every day while he recorded his third album. Unfailingly cheerful, he was a ray of sunshine through the winter months and he had the same sandwich nearly every day, declaring it 'the best sandwich he'd ever had'.

I would have renamed the sandwich in his honour, but you see it's already named after my Grandma Angela. My grandma has made 'egg and onion' for me and my sisters since we were babies, served with bagels on her kitchen table or on open bridge rolls (like mini hot dog rolls, perfect for picking up with one hand while playing bridge) in front of *The Muppet Show* in the living room.

She would never add seeds or the astringent dressing (they're my 'modern' addition), but the gherkins, or simply 'pickles' as she'd call them, are essential.

For the full Grandma Angela experience (passed down from my Great Grandma Cissie), empty the whole fridge onto the table (smoked salmon, fish balls, latkes, chrain, celery sticks, chopped liver, bagels and cream cheese, coleslaw, radishes, cholla, chopped herring and olives) and make everyone eat until they need a lie down. For my niece Angelina and my nephew Jimmy, this feast is as special and as much of a treat as it has always been for me and my sisters. My dad sometimes lays out the same spread, but it's never going to be the same as eating it at Grandma and Big Harry's house, and then falling asleep on their sofa while Grandma strokes my head.

I love having this on the menu at the café, as every time someone orders one it brings back all those memories.

Makes 2

—

3 eggs

2 tbsp good-quality
  mayonnaise

3 spring onions, thinly
  sliced on the diagonal

4 large slices of cholla or
  poppy seed bloomer

1 large gherkin, thinly sliced
  on the diagonal

2 tsp seeds

4 little gem lettuce leaves

Pear Café Dressing
  (see page 227)

flaked sea salt and freshly
  ground black pepper

Cook the eggs according to the 6-minute egg recipe on page 16, but cook them for 8 minutes (you don't want runny yolks).

Peel and, using an egg slicer if you have one, cut each egg into four slices and then into small cubes. Put in a bowl and fold through the mayonnaise and spring onions. Season well.

Spread the egg mixture onto two slices of bread.

Divide the gherkin between the sandwiches. Sprinkle with seeds, drizzle with dressing, and add two lettuce leaves to each sandwich.

Close the sandwich and serve.

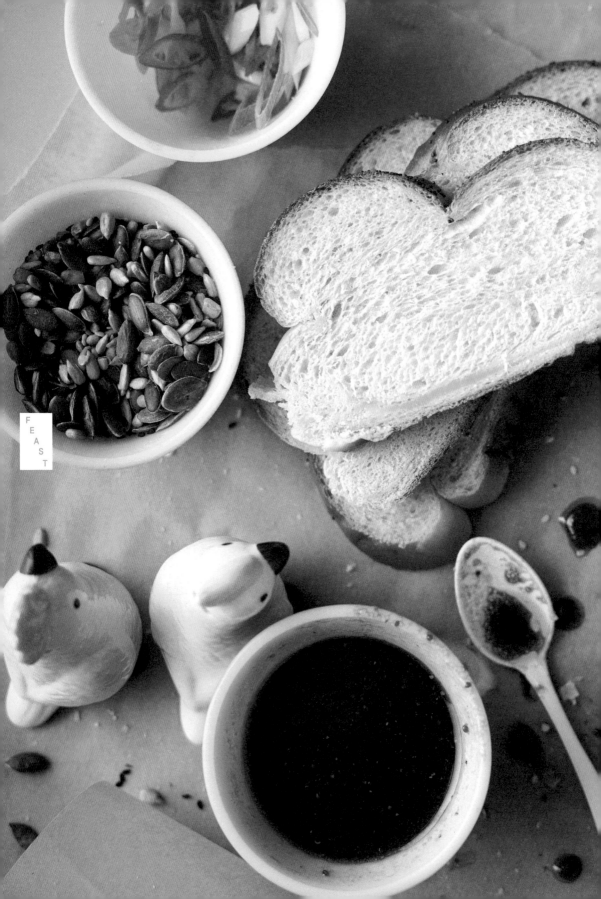

FEAST

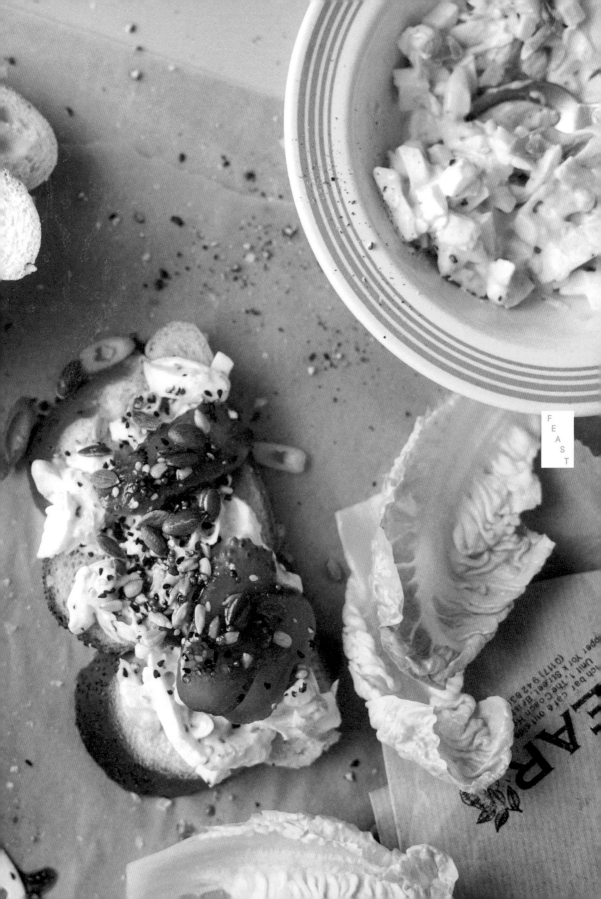

FEAST

How to Batch Cook

Having a well-stocked freezer is the biggest gift you can give to yourself on fast days. Batch cook and freeze whenever you've got the time and inclination for those days when you have precious little of either. If you batch cook and freeze in accurately measured portions, you've basically got yourself 'ready meals' – but you know exactly what's in them. And once your freezer is stocked up, you've got a fast-day-friendly dinner ready to go. A few curries and chillies and some cauliflower rice and you'll be able to get dinner on the table within ten minutes. All you need to do is defrost a portion (or a mixture of portions) in the fridge during the day while you're out and reheat on the hob until piping hot, stirring frequently.

Making these recipes in a big batch will provide endless meals. You can eat them straight away, as is, or change them up into something new. Blitz, add more stock and you have a soup. Add green veg for extra bulk. The list goes on. These recipes are all under 270 kcal per portion, leaving loads of space for making some lush accompaniments. They're also all very cheap (less than £1 a portion), high in protein and #vegan and #glutenfree if you care about such things.

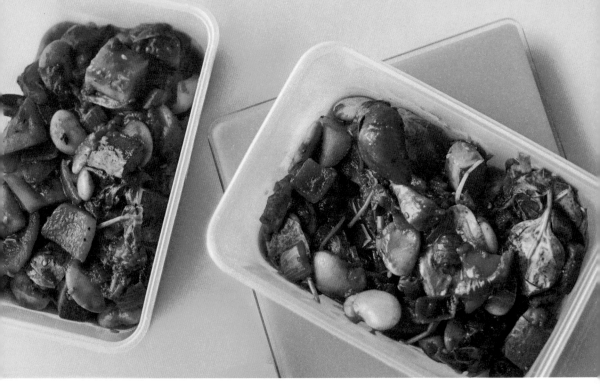

Whenever you cook on a fast day, you have to be really, really accurate. I know, I know — but it's only two days a week. Just do it. Suck it up. Undoubtedly, these calculations are easier and less annoying to do on a feast day when you're not dying to just get the food in your face.

Have a nice session cooking a load of fast-day meals with a glass of wine in hand one evening. You'll be so pleased you did.

You will need
—
digital scales
measuring spoons
a notepad
an online calorie count app
    (like MyFitnessPal)

Method
—

Weigh every ingredient carefully and input the details into your app. This is why you must do it yourself. The size of vegetables will vary, as will the calorie content of tinned tomatoes. Maybe you added something in or took out an ingredient you didn't like. You need to work out YOUR calories for YOUR cooking.

Put a big bowl on the scales and tip the whole lot in. Note the total weight in grams.

Lay out your containers (old plastic takeaway boxes are perfect) and decide how many portions you want to make.

Work out the total number of calories for the entire recipe, then divide up into portions, e.g. whole batch = 600 kcal and 800g. Make 4 portions of 200g each and they'll be 150 kcal each.

Chickpea curry

This chickpea curry freezes brilliantly. Cook up a big batch, divide it up and be ready and prepared for fast days. All you need are some quick accompaniments and you'll have dinner on the table in ten minutes. Seasonal greens, yoghurt and cauliflower rice work perfectly on the side.

Makes 7 portions
—

1 tbsp olive oil

350g chopped onions

large pinch of sea salt

1 tbsp grated root ginger

3 garlic cloves, crushed

1 tsp ground cumin

1 tsp ground coriander

¾ tsp ground turmeric

½ tsp dried chilli flakes

3 cardamom pods,
    lightly crushed

1 cinnamon stick

145g carrot, finely diced

475g chickpeas (drained
    weight), rinsed

2 x 400g tins chopped
    tomatoes

Heat the oil in a large pan. Add the onions and salt and sauté over a medium heat for 15 minutes, until golden. Add the ginger, garlic and spices, and cook for 1 minute, stirring constantly. Pour in 700ml water, add the carrot, chickpeas and tomatoes, then bring to the boil over high heat. Reduce the heat and simmer for 20 minutes, or until the carrot is tender. Remove and discard the cardamom and cinnamon.

Once you've made your curry, follow the How To Batch Cook instructions (page 99) to divide it into portions that can be ready to eat, chilled or frozen.

Variation

A portion of the curry served with 100g of wilted rainbow chard, one portion Kachumber (page 223), 55g of 0% Greek yoghurt and ½ a teaspoon of nigella seeds comes to 207 kcal.

If you're not on a fast day (or you want to eat with someone who's not), brown rice, raita, greens and mango chutney is my favourite combo.

a #batchcookingforfastdays recipe

F
A
S
T

Courgette dhal

198 kcal per portion

Here is a warming and comforting dhal that is gently fragrant and full of goodness. Not to mention that it's incredibly filling, gluten free, can be vegan (if you leave out the egg) and really, really delicious.

Makes 4 portions
—

1 tsp olive oil or coconut oil

120g onion, finely chopped

2 garlic cloves, crushed or very finely chopped

20g root ginger, finely grated

½ tsp garam masala

½ tsp ground cumin

¼ tsp turmeric

½ tsp ground coriander

½ tsp black mustard seeds

¼ tsp curry powder

180g dried red lentils, drained and rinsed well

pinch of flaked sea salt

10g vegetable bouillon powder

400g grated courgettes

1 egg, at room temperature

Garnishes

a few sprigs of coriander

5g finely sliced spring onion

1 lemon wedge

1g toasted sesame seeds or furikake (Japanese rice seasoning)

To make the dhal, heat the oil in a medium pan over a medium heat and cook the onions for 10 minutes, until softened and translucent. Add the garlic and ginger, stir for 1 minute until aromatic, then add the spices. Stir well for about 1 minute, and add a splash of water if the spices are starting to catch. Add the drained lentils and the salt and stir well. Add the vegetable bouillon powder and 500ml boiling water, and cook over medium heat for about 10 minutes, until the lentils turn pale yellow.

Add the grated courgettes and 300ml boiling water. Simmer over a medium heat for a further 10 minutes until the courgettes and lentils are tender. The dhal should be pretty wet, so you may need to add more water if it seems dry.

You can eat it straight away, chill it or freeze it. Whatever your plans for the dhal, you need to divide it up into equal portions as per the instructions on page 99.

Make the 6-minute egg according to instructions on page 16. Peel very carefully, then set to one side. When you've heated up and plated your dhal, hold the egg over your bowl to catch any drips and use a very sharp knife to cut it in half, lengthways. Sit the egg halves on top of your dhal. Garnish with sprigs of coriander, finely sliced spring onion and a wedge of lemon. Sprinkle with sesame seeds or furikake.

Variation

If you're not on a fast day (or you want to eat with someone who's not), wilted buttery greens and naan bread or brown rice is a great combo with the dhal. It's also sublime with fish. The 6-minute eggs are an optional add-on, but really make the dhal into a substantial meal.

F A S T

a #batchcookingforfastdays recipe

Lentil and red pepper chilli

A great base chilli that goes very well with the cauliflower rice (page 16) and can be turned into a variety of other dishes. One way of using this dish is to opt for a Moroccan vibe. Stir mint and parsley through some rice and add coriander, fresh ginger, cinnamon, turmeric, cumin, kale and carrots to the chilli. Serve with a spoon of yoghurt on top.

Makes 7 portions
—

1 tbsp olive oil

180g onion, diced

100g red pepper, deseeded and diced

4 garlic cloves, finely chopped or crushed

2 tsp chilli powder

500g dried green lentils, drained and rinsed

2 x 400g tins chopped tomatoes

1 bay leaf

1 litre vegetable stock (or 10g vegetable bouillon powder dissolved in 1 litre boiling water)

Heat the olive oil in a large pan over medium heat. Add the onion and red pepper and cook for about 8 minutes, until the onion is softened and lightly browned. Stir in the garlic and the chilli and cook for 1 minute. Add the lentils, tomatoes, bay leaf and stock. Bring to the boil over high heat, then lower the heat and simmer, partially covered, for 40 minutes to 1 hour.

Remove the chilli from the heat and discard the bay leaf.

Simply portion up and eat straight away, chill or freeze.

Variation

On feast days serve with avocado, soured cream and rice.

F
A
S
T

a #batchcookingforfastdays recipe

Vegetable, butter bean and smoked paprika stew

187 kcal per portion

There are a million different ways to make ratatouille and this definitely isn't one of them. That's why I haven't called it ratatouille. You'll recognise all those familiar ingredients of the classic Med stew, but this is an altogether simpler affair. To make ratatouille properly, you need loads of oil and loads of time. The vegetables are not cooked separately here, as many recipes for ratatouille call for, as that uses more oil than a fast-day recipe would allow. My version is packed full of veg and, like all these batch-cooking recipes, can be adapted in loads of ways.

Makes 6 portions

—

2 tbsp olive oil

300g aubergine, cut into 1.5cm dice

250g red onions, diced

3 garlic cloves, finely sliced

300g peppers (any colour), deseeded and cut into 1.5cm dice

300g courgettes, cut into 1.5cm dice

2 tsp sweet smoked paprika

2 bay leaves

1 tsp dried oregano

1 x 400g tin plum tomatoes

1 x 400g tin butter beans, drained and rinsed

200g baby spinach

flaked sea salt and freshly ground black pepper, for seasoning

Heat the olive oil in a large saucepan over a medium heat. Add the aubergine, sprinkle with salt and fry for about 5 minutes, until browned. Add the onions and garlic and cook for 4 minutes, stirring regularly, then add the peppers and courgettes. Stir really well and deeply. Cook for a further 5 minutes, stirring regularly, then add the paprika, bay leaves and oregano. Stir well for 1 minute, until aromatic.

Add the tomatoes and their juices, and roughly break them up with the back of your spoon. Mix in the beans and season well with salt and pepper. Add 200ml boiling water, stir, bring to a simmer and cook over a very low heat for 10 minutes. Stir through the spinach and continue to cook for 30 minutes. Taste for seasoning.

You can serve this immediately, but it tastes even better if left in the fridge overnight so the flavours can develop.

Variation

You can serve this with cauliflower rice (see page 16) or whizz up into a soup (add 250ml boiling water and 5g bouillon powder for 12 kcal if you want to stretch it out), top with yoghurt and coriander (30g of 0% Greek yoghurt is 17 kcal), or a little feta and dill (10g of feta is 28 kcal). On a feast day, serve with deep-fried gnocchi and a big dollop of mascarpone on top or lots of crusty bread and some of the Walnut and Basil Pesto (page 236).

F A S T

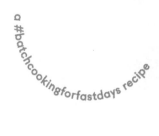

a #batchcookingforfastdays recipe

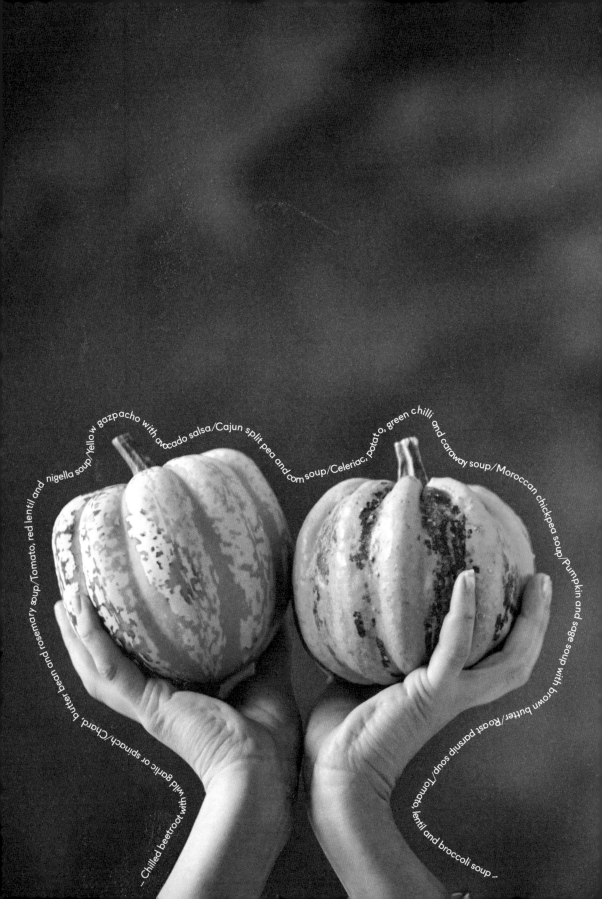

... nigella soup/Yellow gazpacho with avocado salsa/Cajun split pea and corn soup/Celeriac, potato, green chilli and caraway soup/Moroccan chickpea soup/Pumpkin and sage soup with brown butter/Roast parsnip soup/Tomato, lentil and broccoli soup ... Chilled beetroot with wild garlic or spinach/Chard, butter bean and rosemary soup/Tomato, red lentil and

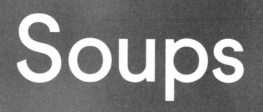

Soups

Tomato, red lentil and nigella soup

Here is a soup that is so easy and quick and made with wholly storecupboard ingredients. That is why it's a perennial favourite at the café. When we've got a lot on, we often make this soup because it needs very little attention and our customers love it. It's by far our most popular soup and we've been making it for years.

Nigella seeds are nothing to do with the wonderful Ms Lawson, by the way. Also called kalonji or black onion seeds, they are very similar to black sesame seeds in appearance although they're not shiny but matt and the blackest of blacks.

Serves 6 generously
—

150g dried red lentils

2 tbsp olive oil

1 medium onion, finely chopped

large pinch of sea salt, plus extra to season

1 tbsp nigella seeds

2 x 400g tins chopped tomatoes

2 tsp vegetable bouillon powder

freshly ground black pepper

First, put your lentils into a large bowl and fill to the top with cold water. Swirl the lentils around with your hand for about 20 seconds – the water will go very cloudy – then gently pour the water out, retaining the lentils in the bowl. Repeat this three or four times, until the water runs nearly clear. Drain.

Heat the olive oil in a saucepan and add the onion and pinch of salt. Cook, over a medium heat for 10 minutes, with the lid on, until the onions are softened. Do not let them brown.

Fill the kettle with water and boil.

When the onions are soft, add the nigella seeds and stir well. Tip the lentils into the pan and then add a splash of boiling water to the lentil bowl to release the last of the lentils. Add this all to the pan along with the tomatoes. Stir really well with a spatula, right to the bottom of the pan, to ensure that no lentils are sticking to the bottom.

Add the bouillon powder and stir well. Pour in 200ml boiling water. Simmer over a medium heat, stirring frequently for about 25 minutes, until the lentils are cooked (they'll go from dark orange to pale yellow and be very soft to bite). Top up with boiling water every now and then if it looks like it is getting too thick.

Use a stick blender to totally blitz the soup until smooth. Add some more water if it's too thick.

Taste for seasoning and serve.

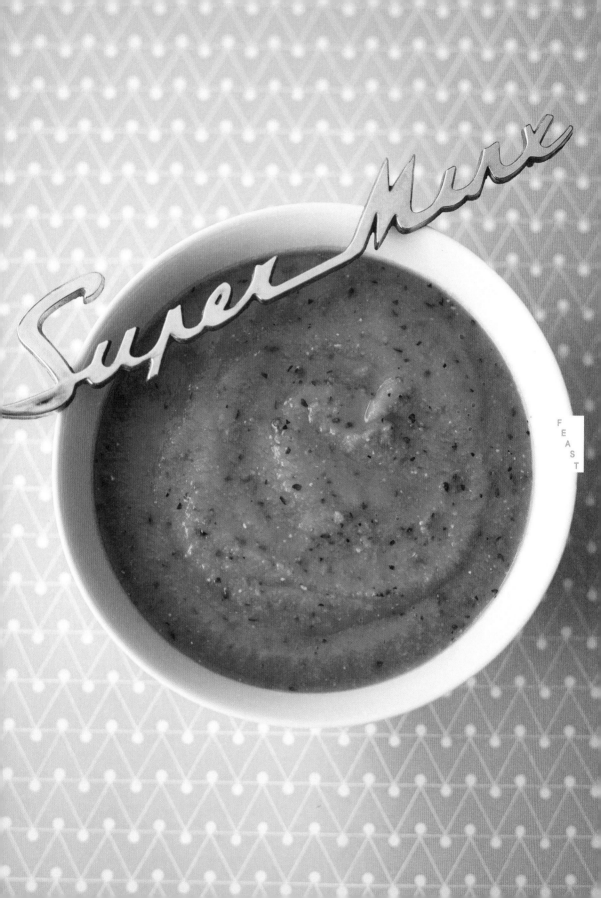

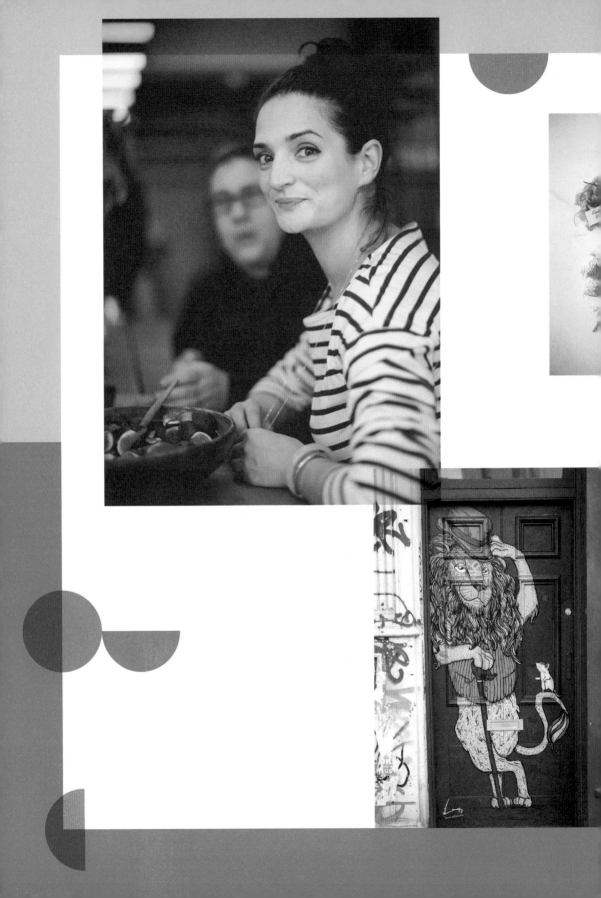

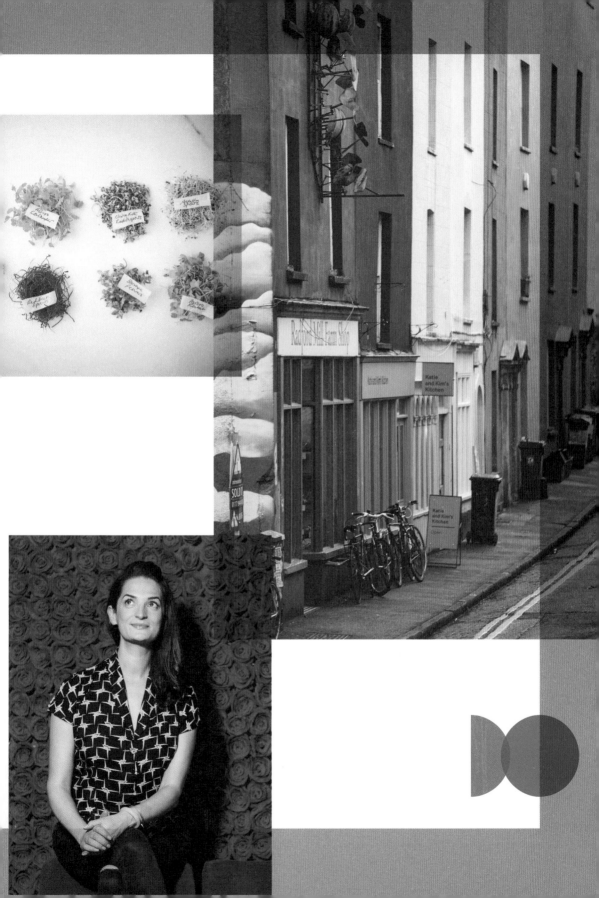

Cajun split pea
and
corn soup

Lots of people are scared of cooking with pulses. Don't be. Not all of them need hours of soaking. Some, like red lentils and yellow split peas, can be simply well washed under cold running water before adding to a soup or stew. Red lentils cook really quickly; yellow split peas are slightly larger, so take a little longer. They're cheap and very nutritious and will sit happily in your storecupboard in well-sealed glass jars for *ages*.

Serves 6

2 tbsp oil

1 large onion, finely diced

2 garlic cloves, crushed or finely diced

1 tsp fine sea salt

1 tbsp Cajun Spice Blend (see page 228)

500g dried yellow split peas

2 litres vegetable stock (made with 4 tsp bouillon powder)

500g frozen sweetcorn

2 tbsp thyme leaves

flaked sea salt and freshly ground black pepper

Heat the oil in a large saucepan and soften the onions and the garlic along with the salt for 10 minutes, over medium-low heat.

Add the Cajun spice blend and the salt, and stir well.

Put the split peas in a bowl and fill with cold water. Swirl the split peas around with your hand for about 20 seconds – the water will go very cloudy – then gently pour the water out, retaining the split peas in the bowl. Repeat this three or four times, until the water runs nearly clear. Drain well.

Add the split peas and the stock to the saucepan and cook for 20 minutes over a medium heat.

Stir in the sweetcorn and cook for a further 45 minutes, until all the split peas are tender.

Add the thyme, then use a stick blender, or transfer to a blender, and blitz until smooth.

Taste for seasoning and serve.

Moroccan chickpea soup

This makes a huge batch of soup and it freezes well. The recipe involves quite a bit of chopping, so do it now and benefit in the future.

Serves 10

—

2 tsp olive oil

3 celery sticks, finely diced

3 carrots, finely diced

2 onions, finely diced

3 garlic cloves,
    finely chopped

2 tsp ground cumin

2 tsp ground coriander

1 tsp ground ginger

1 tsp ground cinnamon

1 tsp Turkish chilli flakes

1 tsp smoked paprika

2 tsp date syrup

4 x 400g tins chopped
    tinned tomatoes

2 x 400g tins chickpeas,
    drained and rinsed

4 tsp bouillon powder

juice of ¼ a lemon

fresh coriander, roughly
    chopped

flaked sea salt and freshly
    ground black pepper

Heat the olive oil in a pan, add the celery, carrots, onions, garlic, salt and pepper and cook for 10 minutes over a medium–low heat, until softened. Add all of the spices, stir, and cook for 2 minutes. Fill the kettle and boil.

Add the date syrup, tomatoes, chickpeas and bouillon powder and cover with boiling water. Simmer over a medium heat for 20 minutes, until the chickpeas are soft.

Use a stick blender to semi-blend the soup until the desired consistency (I like it pretty chunky). Check for seasoning.

To serve, stir through the lemon juice and roughly chopped coriander.

FEAST

Yellow gazpacho with avocado salsa

This gazpacho is a refreshing treat and looks great made with yellow tomatoes, but obviously you can use regular red ones if you prefer. It is best made at the height of summer when tomatoes are properly ripe and full of flavour. I like to make it in the morning, chill it well and have a couple of small bowls throughout the day, then use up the rest of the ingredients in a salad for dinner.

Serves 2
—

3 garlic cloves

60ml sherry vinegar

¼ cup chopped coriander

¼ tsp Tabasco

½ tsp ground cumin

200g yellow tomatoes

140g yellow pepper, deseeded

100g cucumber, deseeded

30g ripe avocado flesh

For the avocado salsa

4g red onion, finely diced

20g cherry tomatoes, finely diced

30g ripe avocado flesh, finely diced

flaked sea salt, to taste

F
A
S
T

Simply blend all the ingredients, except the avocado salsa, until totally smooth in your food processor or blender, and chill for at least 3 hours. Taste for seasoning.

Just before serving, combine the ingredients for the avocado salsa in a small bowl.

To serve, ladle the soup into a bowl and top with the salsa.

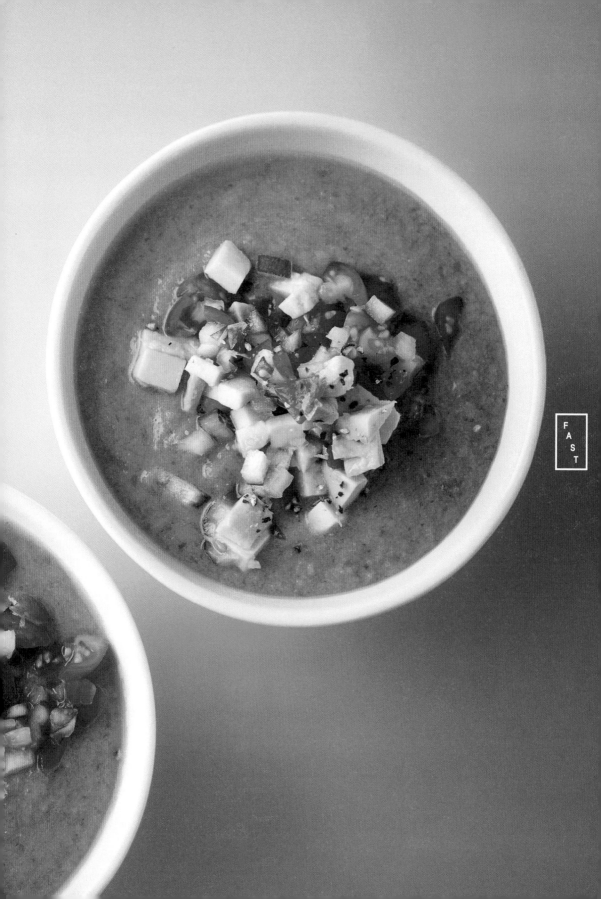

Chard, butter bean and rosemary soup

It's the added garnishes that make this soup. As the heat releases the fragrance of the lemon and rosemary, the Parmesan starts to melt into the soup. Finish with a load of fresh black pepper and you've made a great soup even more delicious. If you can't find rainbow chard, spring greens or kale make a good alternative. The soup keeps well in the fridge for up to three days and freezes well, too.

On a feast day, I'd chargrill a piece of good bread, drizzle it with your best olive oil and rub it with a garlic clove. Serve half submerged in the soup.

Serves 2

—

1 tsp olive oil

100g carrot, finely diced

100g onions, finely diced

1 garlic clove, crushed

50g leek, sliced into
    fine rings

2 tsp rosemary, very finely
    chopped

¼ tsp dried chilli flakes

1 tbsp sherry vinegar

500ml vegetable
    stock (made with
    10g vegetable
    bouillon powder)

140g tinned butter beans,
    drained and rinsed

140g rainbow chard,
    stalks chopped and
    leaves sliced into ribbons

flaked sea salt and freshly
    ground black pepper

For the garnish

1 tsp finely grated lemon zest

10g Parmesan, very
    finely grated

Heat the oil in a medium pan, add the carrot, onions, garlic and leek, season with salt and pepper. Cover and cook over a medium heat for 10 minutes, until the onion is translucent and the carrot is softened.

Add 1 teaspoon rosemary, the chilli flakes and the sherry vinegar, and cook over medium heat for 1 minute.

Add the stock, butter beans and chard stalks, and cook for 5 minutes over a low heat. Add the chard leaves and warm through for a couple of minutes. Plate up. Sprinkle with lemon zest, Parmesan and the remaining rosemary. Season well with black pepper. Serve.

F
A
S
T

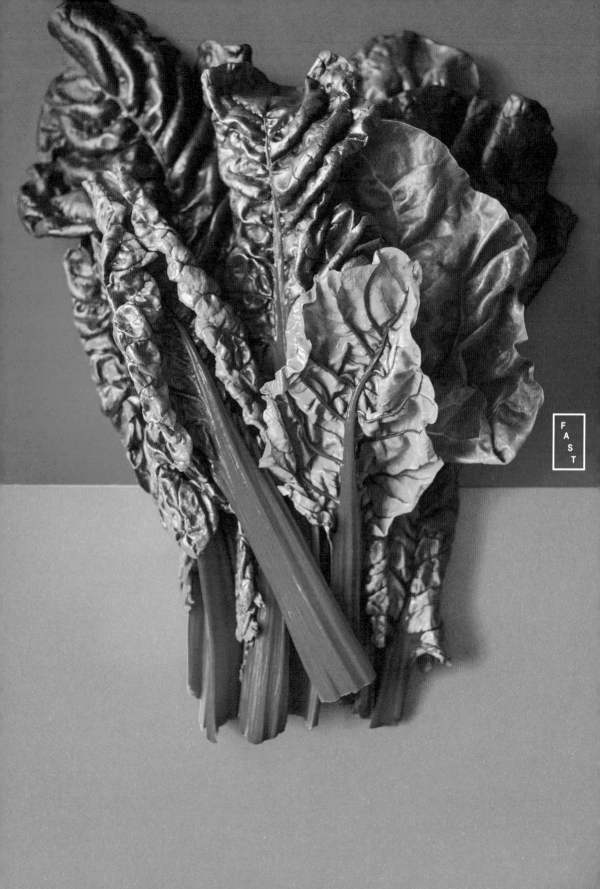

Chilled beetroot soup
with wild garlic or spinach

This recipe is super-quick, full of goodness and really cheap. Frankly, what more could you want?

It's also made with ingredients that are really easy to find and it keeps well. It's lush both hot and chilled, so is great all year round.

The downside is you will almost certainly splatter your clothes with beetroot juice, so don't wear white. I wore white.

I first made this with wild garlic I picked myself. It's all over the place for a few weeks each spring (look in damp wooded areas and follow the smell of garlic). But once it's gone, you can make it with baby spinach and some chives and it's equally delicious.

Serves 2
—

1 x 250g packet cooked beetroot

20g wild garlic leaves, roughly torn (or baby spinach plus 1 tablespoon finely chopped chives)

250ml hot vegetable stock (made with 1 tsp bouillon powder)

flaked sea salt and freshly ground black pepper

For the garnish

1 tsp lemon juice

15g Greek yoghurt

a few coriander or dill leaves

Simply open the pack of beetroot and tip the whole lot into a jug blender. I use a Vitamix, but a Nutribullet or any other blender would be fine. The stronger the engine, the quicker and smoother it will be.

Add the wild garlic, stock, salt and pepper and blend until totally smooth.

Taste for seasoning. You can either eat it straight away (it should still be hot enough from the hot stock) or chill and serve cold.

Before serving, mix the lemon juice and yoghurt together, adding a tiny splash of cold water if it's too thick, and drizzle on top of the soup. Garnish with the herbs. Eat.

F
A
S
T

Tomato, lentil and broccoli soup

178 kcal per portion

Swapping some of the bulk of the lentils with the far lower-calorie broccoli cuts down the calorie count hugely.

Serves 5

—

1 tsp extra-virgin olive oil

120g onions, finely diced

2 tsp Turkish chilli flakes

200g dried red lentils, drained and well rinsed

60g broccoli, chopped

2 x 400g tins chopped tomatoes

flaked sea salt and freshly ground black pepper

Heat the oil in a pan and add the onions, chilli flakes and a good pinch of salt. Stir well and cook over a medium heat for a few minutes, until the onions start to colour. Fill the kettle and boil.

Add the lentils and broccoli and stir well. Cook for 2 minutes over a low heat, stirring regularly.

Add the tinned tomatoes along with 500ml boiling water, bring to the boil over medium-high heat, then reduce the heat to medium-low and cook for about 15–20 minutes until the lentils are tender. Remove from the heat and use a stick blender to purée. Season to taste and serve.

F
A
S
T

Pumpkin and sage soup with brown butter

This is a silky, deeply fragrant, indulgent soup. The roasted garlic gives a wonderful depth of flavour, but the real stars of the show are the toppings — crème fraîche, sage, brown butter and pumpkin seeds. You could serve this soup without them, but you'd really be missing out.

Serves 4

——

1 head of garlic, whole

2 tbsp olive oil

1 small leek, finely sliced and well rinsed in warm water

1 medium onion, finely chopped

10 sage leaves

350g peeled and roughly cubed pumpkin or butternut squash

2 tsp vegetable bouillon powder

¼ tsp smoked salt

1 bay leaf

1 x 400g tin butter beans, drained and rinsed

freshly ground black pepper

For the topping

2 tbsp Brown Butter (see page 234)

6 small sage leaves

4 heaped tsp crème fraîche

4 tsp pumpkin seeds, toasted

To serve

4 slices of sourdough bread

1 garlic clove, peeled and cut in half lengthways

olive oil, for drizzling

Preheat the oven to 180°C/350°F/Gas mark 4. Slice a quarter off the top of the garlic head and put the rest on the centre of a 25cm square of foil. Drizzle over 1 tablespoon olive oil and wrap the foil up tightly around the garlic. Place on a baking sheet in the middle of the oven and roast for 30–45 minutes, until it feels really squishy. Remove, carefully (it will be hot!) loosen the foil and leave until cool enough to handle. Fill the kettle and boil.

Squeeze the roasted garlic cloves out of the bulb into a large pan placed over medium heat. Add the remaining tablespoon of olive oil to the pan with the garlic, along with the leek and the onion, and stir well. Cook for 5 minutes, stirring regularly, until the leek starts to soften.

Stir in the sage and squash and cook for 2 minutes over a medium heat. Add the bouillon powder and enough boiling water to cover the vegetables. Season well, add the bay leaf, stir, and bring to the boil. Add the beans, cover and simmer over a low heat for about 20 minutes, until the squash is tender.

Remove the pan from the heat and using a stick blender to blitz until smooth (or leave semi-chunky if you prefer). Add more boiling water if it's too thick. Taste for seasoning.

To make the topping, heat the brown butter in a pan over a medium heat. Fry the sage leaves for 30 seconds, until crisp.

Toast or grill your sourdough bread and rub both sides with the cut side of the garlic. Drizzle with olive oil.

Divide the soup into bowls and add a drizzle of the sage brown butter. Add a big dollop of crème fraîche and a sprinkle of the fried sage leaves. Finish with a few toasted pumpkin seeds.

Serve each bowl with the garlicky bread.

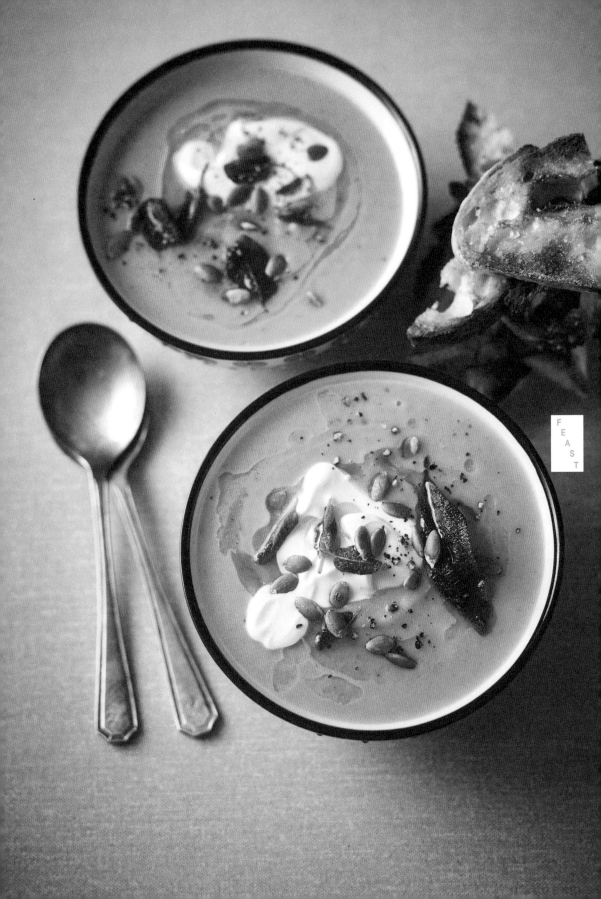

Celeriac, potato, green chilli and caraway soup

This recipe was created by Marinella, one of the first members of Team Pear Café. She's Italian and grew up in rural Tuscany, but has also travelled extensively and has an excellent understanding of flavour, inspired by world cooking. She definitely left her mark on the café and we think of her often. This soup is one of the only times I ever use green chillies.

Serves 4–6

---

2 tbsp olive oil

1 medium onion, finely sliced

2 garlic cloves, finely sliced

1 green medium-sized chilli, finely chopped

1 tsp caraway seeds, plus extra to serve

1 large celeriac, peeled and diced

1 tbsp vegetable bouillon powder

1kg potatoes, peeled and diced

flaked sea salt and freshly ground black pepper

extra-virgin olive oil, for drizzling

Heat the olive oil in a pan, add the onion, garlic, chilli and caraway seeds and a pinch of salt, and cook for 10 minutes over a medium-low heat, until softened. Add the celeriac, stir well and continue to cook for 10 minutes.

Add the bouillon powder with enough boiling water to cover the vegetables, and cook for 15 minutes.

Add the potatoes, pour over more water to cover, and cook for about 35–45 minutes, until all the vegetables are tender.

Use a stick blender to blend the soup until creamy and totally smooth. Season to taste.

Serve with a drizzle of extra-virgin olive oil and some caraway seeds on top.

Roast parsnip soup

All you need to do for this recipe is tumble all the veg together in one big tray, roast, and then blitz. Simple and delicious.

Serves 4
—

1kg parsnips, peeled and roughly chopped

2 tomatoes, quartered

1 red onion, peeled and chopped into wedges

1 tbsp black mustard seeds

2 tbsp extra-virgin olive oil

30ml balsamic vinegar

2 tsp vegetable bouillon powder

flaked sea salt and freshly ground black pepper

Preheat the oven to 180°C/350°F/Gas mark 4.

Toss all the ingredients apart from the balsamic vinegar and vegetable bouillon powder together in a large bowl, then spread out in a roasting tin.

Roast for about 45 minutes to 1 hour, until the parsnips are golden brown and the edges are starting to char.

Tip into a large pan and deglaze the roasting tin with the balsamic vinegar and a splash of water. Pour this into the pan, too.

Add the vegetable bouillon powder, topping up with boiling water to cover the vegetables, then use a stick blender to blitz to a smooth consistency.

F
E
A
S
T

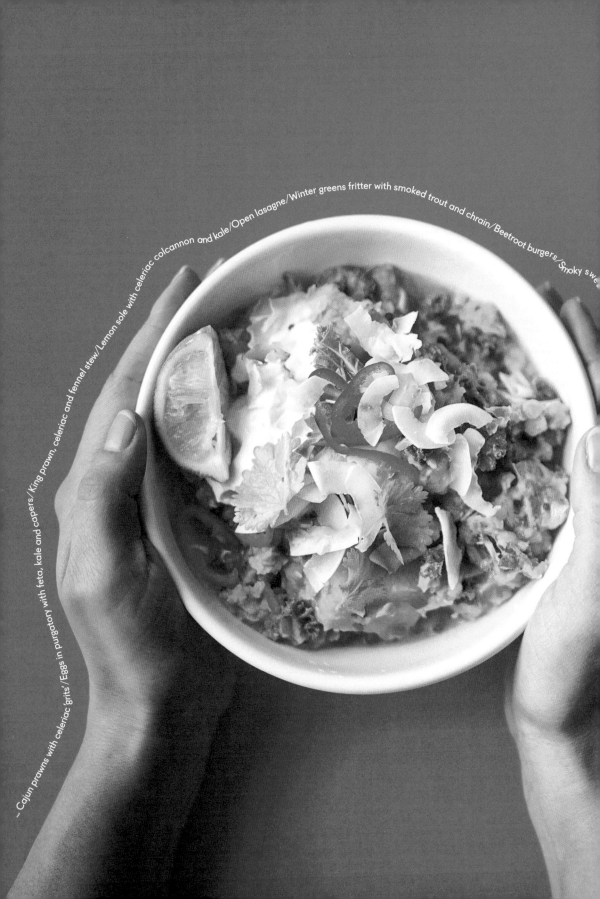

... Cajun prawns with celeriac grits/Eggs in purgatory with feta, kale and capers/King prawn, celeriac and fennel stew/Lemon sole with celeriac colcannon and kale/Open lasagne/Winter greens fritter with smoked trout and chrain/Beetroot burgers/Smoky swe

Weeknight Dinners

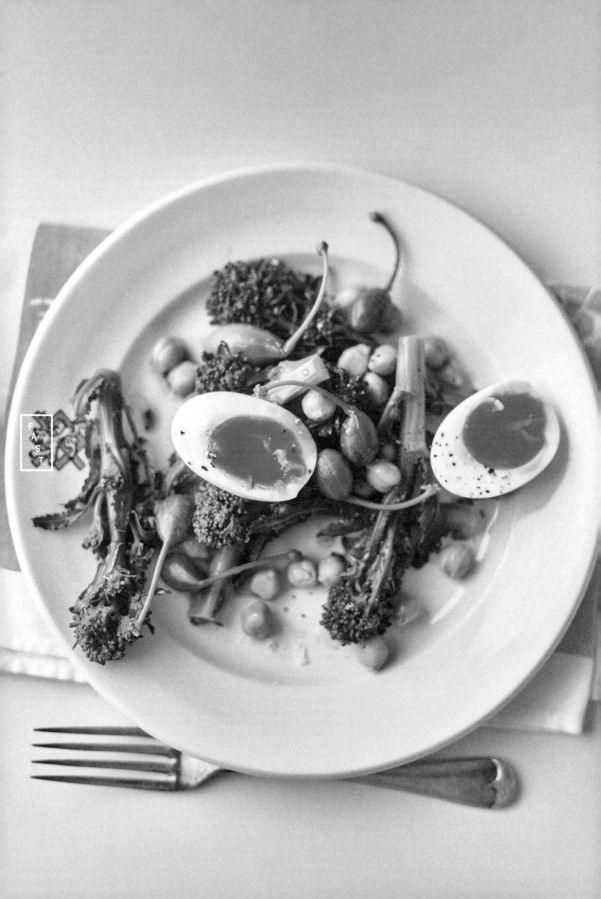

Purple sprouting broccoli, egg, caper berries and chickpeas

172 kcal
per portion

Here is a great base recipe — storecupboard ingredients served up with seasonal greens. In this case I'm using purple sprouting broccoli, but it also works well with spring greens, kale or courgette ribbons. Keep a jar of caper berries in your fridge (they're a great addition to salads), and make sure you've always got a few tins of chickpeas and good eggs to hand. You've got the start of a million great meals.

Serves 1

—

80g purple sprouting broccoli, trimmed

6-minute egg (see page 16), cut in half

25g caper berries

35g tinned chickpeas, drained and rinsed (use the remaining chickpeas for Hummous, page 216 or in the Sweet Potato, Chickpea and Kale Salad on page 62)

¼ tsp extra-virgin olive oil

2 tsp sherry vinegar

flaked sea salt and freshly ground black pepper

Bring a pan of salted water to the boil and gently lower the broccoli in, stalk end first. Cook for 4–5 minutes, until cooked but still *al dente*. Drain well.

Arrange the cooked broccoli, egg, caper berries and chickpeas on a plate.

Dress with the extra-virgin olive oil and the sherry vinegar.

Season well and serve.

F
A
S
T

Winter sunshine salad

In the depths of winter, everything can get a bit heavy. You're swaddled in thick clothes and downing soup and stews like nobody's business just to keep warm. The central heating and cold wind can leave you feeling dried out and crusty as hell.

You and your skin need a vitamin boost, and a huge bowl of crunchy, brightly coloured salad full of vitamins C and E is coming to the rescue. Chomp your way through the nuts, seeds and veg and you'll feel like a million bucks.

If you want to serve it the next day, keep the dressing separate until you're ready to eat.

This goes really well with salmon or tuna (great for adding omega-3 fatty acids) and is also lush with feta sprinkled on top.

Serves 2
—

1 bunch of kale, prepared according to instructions on page 17, roughly chopped

100g red cabbage, finely sliced

2 carrots, cut into fine matchsticks or grated

2 large handfuls of flat-leaf parsley leaves, roughly chopped

1 large or 2 small raw beetroot, peeled and cut into fine matchsticks or grated

1 apple, cut into 1cm dice

½ red onion, cut into very fine dice

flaked sea salt and freshly ground black pepper

For the dressing
2 tbsp olive oil
2 tbsp apple cider vinegar
1 tsp tahini
finely grated zest of ½ lemon
1 garlic clove, crushed
1 tbsp maple syrup

To garnish
small handful of toasted walnuts
small handful of toasted pecans
1 tbsp hemp seeds
1 tsp linseeds (flaxseeds)
1 tbsp pumpkin seeds

Mix all the dressing ingredients up in a jar and shake really well.

Pour into a large salad bowl and tip in all the salad ingredients. Season. Use your hands to toss everything together, massaging the dressing into the salad for 2 minutes.

Top with the nuts and seeds, and serve.

Tahini noodles with greens and 6-minute egg

On the table in about 15 minutes, this is ideal weeknight fodder. If you want to increase the serving size to two, make the marinated tofu from the recipe on page 146 and nestle it on top of the noodles with the egg.

Serves 1
—

100g greens
(such as cavolo nero,
chard, kale or pak choi)
1 tbsp vegetable oil
1 egg
1 x 300g packet straight-to-
wok udon noodles
1 tbsp soy sauce
1 tbsp Tahini Noodle
Dressing (page 229)
1 heaped tbsp sauerkraut

To garnish
furikake (Japanese rice
seasoning) or Pear
Café Seed Blend
(see page 227)
mixed seaweed flakes,
optional

Trim the greens and chop if necessary. Rinse in water and shake dry.

Get the water on to boil your 6-minute egg (see page 16).

When the water for the egg is boiling, heat the vegetable oil in a wok or large pan.

Put the egg into the water, following the 6-minute egg recipe on page 16. Remember to set your timer.

Back to the wok, when the oil is hot, add the noodles. Toss in the oil and stir-fry over medium-high heat for 1 minute. Add the greens, stir-fry for 1 minute, then add the soy sauce. Keep stir-frying for another 1 minute or so, until the timer goes off for the egg.

Tip into a serving bowl. Drain the egg and blast it with cold water from the tap for a few seconds so that the egg is cool enough to peel. Tap the shell all over, then peel the egg.

Dress the noodles with the Tahini Noodle Dressing.

Hold the egg over the noodles and carefully cut it in half. (Be careful not to let the yolk go on your fingers, as it'll be very hot.) Sit the egg on the noodles. Add the sauerkraut on the side, and scatter the furikake and seaweed, if using, on top.

F
E
A
S
T

Roasted romanesco and asparagus with lime and coriander dressing

Swap the veggies around depending on what's in season; the tahini and lime dressing loves them all equally. Alternative veg possibilities include regular cauliflower, new potatoes, shallots, spring onions or sweet potato.

Serve with a little gem salad and be sure to include some seeds or nuts for crunch and protein. This is also great served cold.

Serves 2

---

1 head of romanesco, broken into florets

1 red onion, cut into wedges

6 asparagus spears

extra-virgin olive oil

flaked sea salt and freshly ground black pepper

For the dressing

a handful of coriander, chopped

juice of 1 lime

1 tbsp tahini

4 tbsp olive oil

1½ tbsp sherry vinegar

1 tsp runny honey

For the toppings

natural yoghurt

pomegranate molasses

Pear Café Seed Blend, see page 227)

toasted almonds or hazelnuts, roughly chopped

wild garlic oil (see page 237) or finely chopped chives

pea shoots or rocket

Preheat the oven to 200°C/400°F/Gas mark 6. Toss the romanesco, onion and asparagus in a little extra-virgin olive oil and season with salt and pepper. Roast the romanesco and onion on a lined baking tray for 10 minutes, then add the asparagus and cook until everything is nicely charred at the edges.

Whisk all the dressing ingredients in a bowl. When the veg comes out of the oven, allow them to cool slightly. Lightly splatter the dressing all over, top the veg with your choice of toppings and season well.

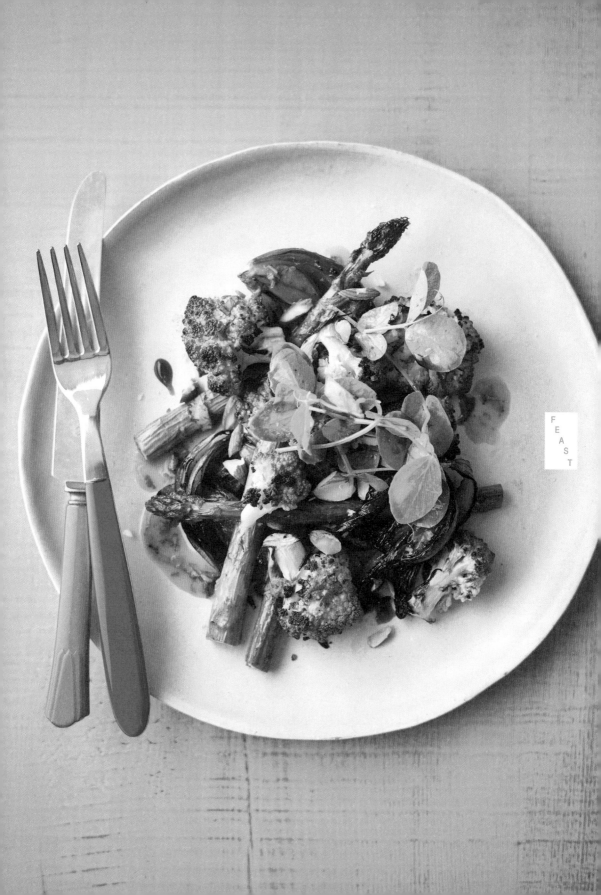

FEAST

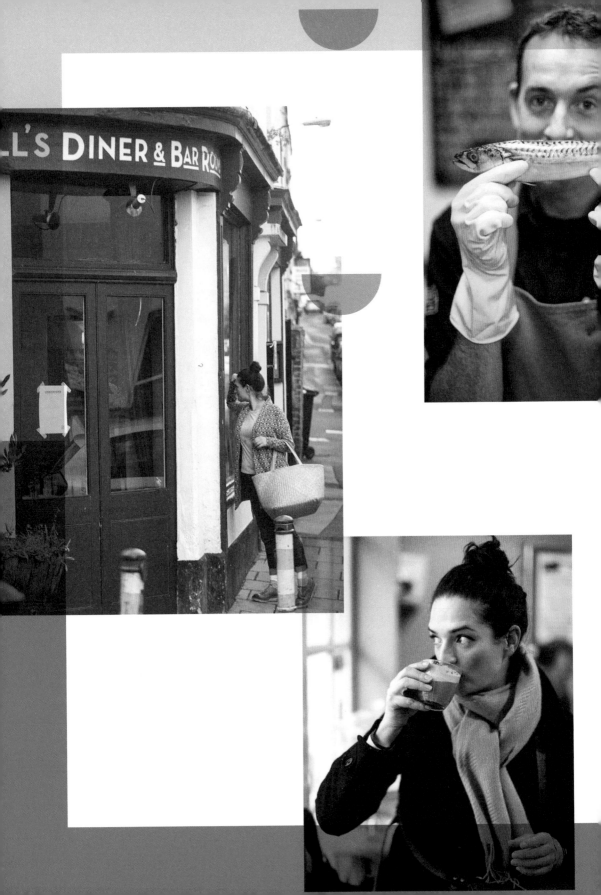

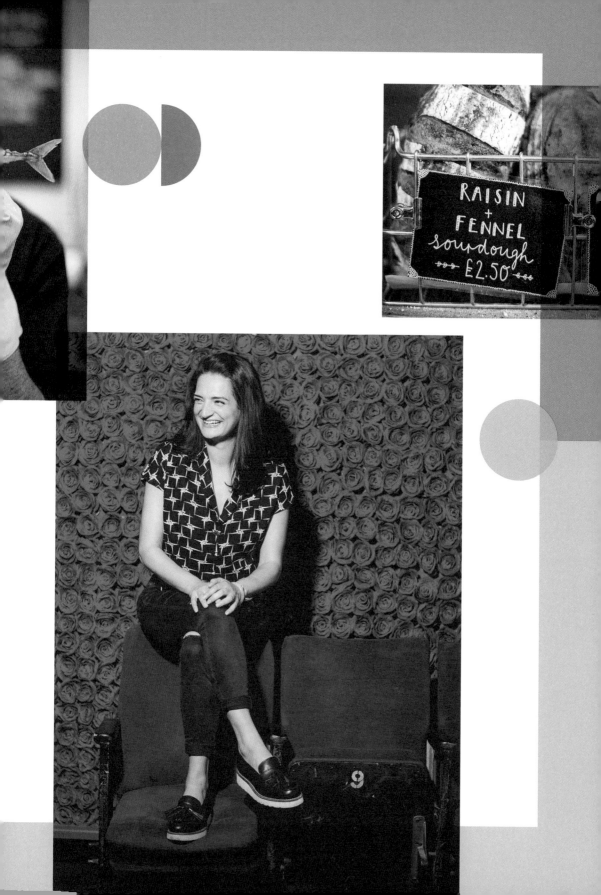

RAISIN
+
FENNEL
sourdough
•≫• £2.50 •≪•

Roasted broccoli

ᵃnd

smoked tofu salad

This makes a delicious, filling, nutritious dinner but also travels really well and is great served cold as a packed lunch. The avocado will go brown if it's exposed to air for too long, so if you're not eating the salad straight away, pack the avocado separately and peel and cube it just before serving.

Serves 2

1 head of broccoli

2 banana shallots, or
    4 regular shallots, sliced

1 tbsp olive oil, plus extra
    for drizzling

zest and juice of 1 lemon

1 tbsp finely grated Parmesan

1 x 200g packet ready-to-eat
    smoked tofu, cubed

4 pickled baby beetroots,
    roughly chopped

2 large handfuls of prepared
    kale (see page 17)

1 ripe avocado

flaked sea salt and freshly
    ground black pepper

To serve

2 tbsp Golden Amazing
    Sauce (see page 220)

a large pinch of China rose
    radish sprouts

1 heaped tbsp toasted
    pumpkin seeds

Preheat the oven to 180°C/350°F/Gas mark 4.

Peel and thickly slice the broccoli stalk (most of the goodness is in the stalk – don't waste it) and break the head into florets.

Put the broccoli and shallots in a bowl, drizzle with olive oil and sprinkle with salt and pepper. Tip into a baking tray lined with baking parchment. Set the bowl you used to one side.

Roast in the oven for 20 minutes, until charred. Tip the contents of the tin back into the reserved bowl. Grate over the lemon zest and squeeze the juice, add the 1 tablespoon of olive oil and the Parmesan.

Add in the smoked tofu, beetroot and kale. Slice the avocado in half, remove the stone and slice the flesh into cubes. Add this to the bowl and mix well. Transfer to a serving bowl.

To serve, drizzle with the Golden Amazing Sauce and garnish with sprouts and pumpkin seeds.

Twenty-minute cheat's tagine

This is a perfect midweek dinner. Really quick and full of goodness – and as both butternut squashes and onions are pretty hardy and keep for ages, you can whip it up without having to go and buy any fresh produce. It could also definitely be multiplied and frozen in portions. I love the yoghurt on top, but it's fine to leave it off if you prefer to keep the tagine vegan.

Serves 2

—

glug of olive oil

1 small onion, finely chopped

300g butternut squash, peeled and diced

2 tsp harissa

1 x 400g tin chickpeas, drained and rinsed

1 cinnamon stick

1 tsp ground cumin

1 tsp vegetable bouillon powder

flaked sea salt and freshly ground black pepper

To serve

natural yoghurt or Greek yoghurt

fresh coriander and mint leaves and chive flowers (if in season)

cooked rice, couscous or cauliflower rice (see page 16)

Heat the olive oil in a pan and add the onion and a pinch of salt. Fry for 10 minutes, over a medium heat, until soft and translucent, then add the squash. Stir in the harissa and cook for a couple of minutes, then add the chickpeas, cinnamon, cumin, 150ml boiling water and the bouillon powder.

Put a lid on and simmer over a low heat for 10 minutes until the squash is tender. Season well.

Garnish with yoghurt, lots of coriander and mint leaves and, if they're in season, chive flowers.

Serve with rice, couscous or cauliflower rice (see page 16).

F
E
A
S
T

Sweet potato, lentil, kale and coconut curry

A lentil and kale curry? This might be the most hippy curry ever (hell, chuck some hemp seeds on top and give it a crown), but it's also one of my favourites. Like all curries, it's even better the next day. It's nutritious, filling and delicious and you can just as easily make it for ten as you can for two, so it's a great one for informal suppers with family or mates. Do the garnishing with a little extra effort and as much panache as you can muster. It looks really great once it's all topped and, I think you'll agree, even better next to a cold beer.

Serves 6

—

2 tbsp vegetable oil

125g chopped onion

4 garlic cloves, crushed

¼ tsp freshly grated root ginger

2 tsp mustard seeds

1 tsp cumin seeds

1 tsp turmeric

¼ tsp chilli powder

450g dried red lentils, drained and rinsed

1 medium sweet potato, cut into 2.5cm cubes

2 x 400g tins chopped tomatoes

1 x 400ml tin coconut milk

2 generous pinches of flaked sea salt

2 large handfuls of prepared kale (see page 17)

a handful of coriander, stalks finely chopped and leaves roughly chopped

1 tsp very finely diced red chilli

To serve

1 small handful coconut flakes, toasted

1 tsp cumin seeds, toasted

lime wedges

Greek yoghurt

1 red chilli, sliced

Heat the vegetable oil in a pan and add the onion. Cook over a low heat for about 15 minutes, until really soft and slightly golden. This will really bring out all the sweet flavour of the onion. Add the garlic and ginger and cook for 1 minute over a medium heat. Stir through the spices and cook for 2 minutes, then add the lentils. Stir. Add the sweet potato, tomatoes, coconut milk and 300ml boiling water and stir well.

Turn the heat right down and simmer very gently for 30 minutes, until the lentils are cooked and the sweet potato is tender. Remember to stir deeply and often during the cooking time so that the lentils don't stick to the bottom of the pan.

Add in the kale and top up with a bit more water if the curry seems too dry. The kale should cook adequately within a couple of minutes – you want it wilted but still *al dente*.

Remove from the heat. Season well and add in a good handful of the chopped coriander and the fresh chilli.

Plate up, top with the coconut flakes, cumin seeds and the remaining coriander and a wedge of lime. Serve with yoghurt and extra fresh chilli for people to add if they want to.

This is mega filling and doesn't really need additional carbs, but a roti might be good to mop up the sauce.

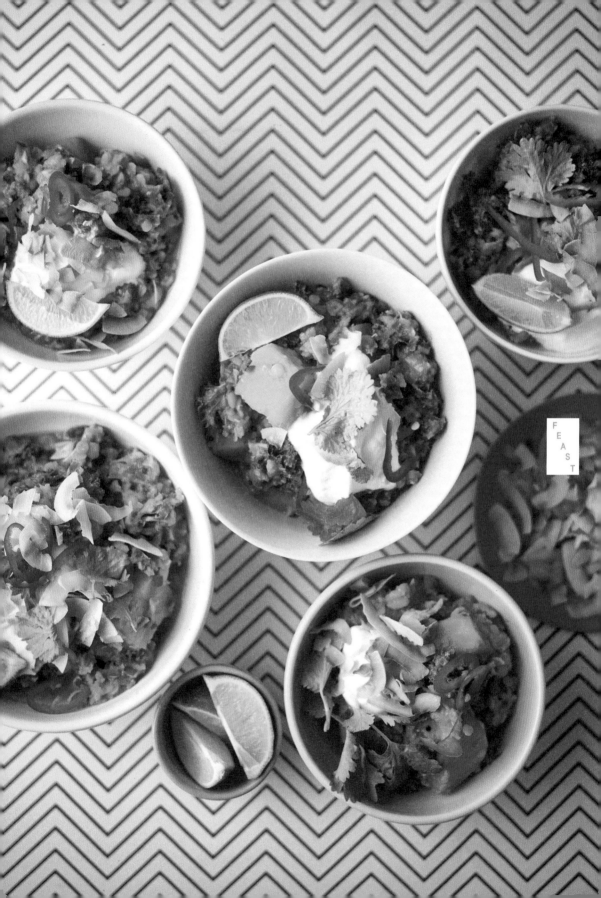

FEAST

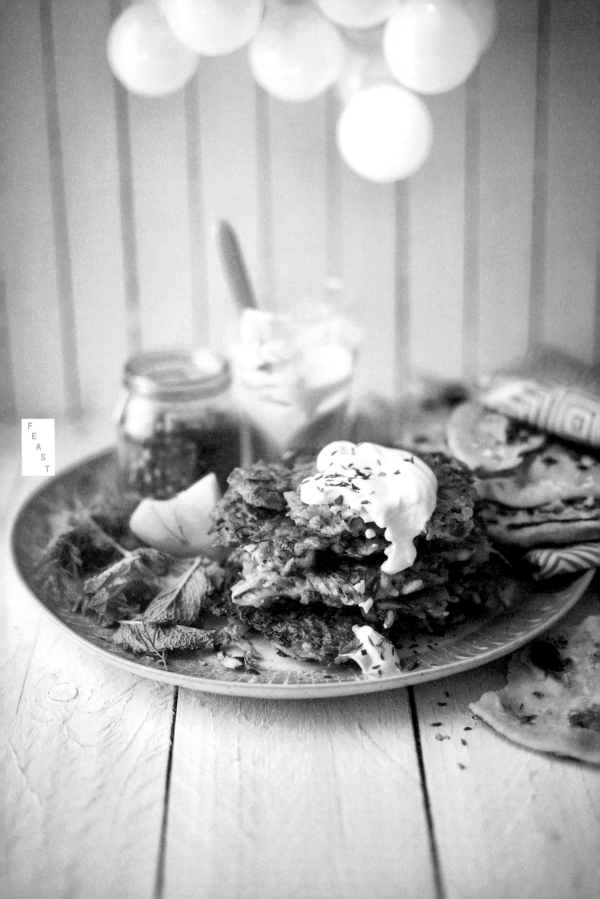

Root veg and halloumi fritters with frying-pan flatbread

These are inspired by the courgette and halloumi fritters I ate at Bells Diner in Bristol. A quintessential Antipodean brunch dish, usually served with poached eggs, they also make a great light supper dish, eaten in the sunshine with a glass of wine. Don't worry, I checked.

The flatbreads are a bit of a revelation. I swear they take less than ten minutes from start to finish, and you don't need to wait for the mixture to rise or even knead the dough for that long. They are ridiculously easy to make. Here, the flatbreads complement the fritters, the sharp lemon juice-dressed slaw and the crispy green salad – but they're also ace as used on page 170, like a kind of cheat's mega-quick pizza base. Feel free to mix a teaspoon of sesame or nigella seeds into the dough mix if you want to jazz up the flatbreads.

Serves 2 as a main, or 4 as a starter depending on size of the fritters

—

For the flatbreads

175g plain flour, plus extra for dusting

generous pinch of salt

olive oil, for frying

flaked sea salt, for sprinkling

Recipe continues overleaf

First, put the grated veg in a colander and squeeze as dry as you can. Leave to drain while you get on with the rest of the recipe.

Next, make the flatbreads. In a large bowl, add the flour, 100ml water and pinch of salt. Mix until the dough is just sticking together, but not too moist. Put the dough on a floured work surface and knead for 3 minutes. Roll the dough into a log and cut it into four portions.

Flour a rolling pin and roll each portion of the dough out into a 2–4mm thick round.

Heat a large frying pan and coat the bottom with olive oil. Set over a medium-high heat. Fry the flatbreads, one at a time, for 1 minute or so on the first side until the edges have hardened and the surface starts to bubble. Flip it. Cook the second side for another minute or so until it is bubbly and golden brown. Slide onto a plate and sprinkle with sea salt.

Cover loosely with a clean tea towel while you cook the remaining flatbreads. Once they're all done, put to one side until everything else is ready.

Wipe out your pan.

For the fritters, tip all the drained veg into a bowl and add the halloumi, herbs and caraway seeds. Season well with plenty of black pepper and a small pinch of sea salt.

For the fritters

200g mixture of coarsely grated carrot, parsnip and beetroot (approximately 1 carrot, 1 parsnip, 1 medium beetroot)

100g halloumi, coarsely grated

2 tbsp finely chopped mint, plus a few whole leaves for garnishing

2 tbsp finely chopped dill, plus a few whole sprigs for garnishing

¼ tbsp toasted caraway seeds, plus a little for sprinkling

2 eggs, beaten

3 tbsp plain flour (optional)

vegetable, sunflower or grapeseed oil, for frying

flaked sea salt and freshly ground black pepper

To serve

Greek Yoghurt

Turkish chilli flakes

lemon wedges

Add the eggs and mix well. Next, add the flour, if using, spoonful by spoonful, and mix well. You're looking to make a dry enough mixture that will form a firm fritter but will still stay together. You might not need all the flour, or you may need a little more.

Heat the oil in the pan over a medium heat. Form the mixture into six fritters and fry for approximately 5 minutes on each side, until golden brown and hot all the way through (poke the tip of a sharp knife into the centre of one – there should be no wet batter). If the fritters brown too quickly, turn the heat right down to low.

Take off the heat and serve your fritters topped with the Greek Yoghurt, a sprinkle of sea salt, a pinch of Turkish chilli flakes, the remaining fresh herbs and the lemon wedges and flatbreads alongside.

I like to also balance the fried fritters and bread with a sharp dressed slaw and a crispy green salad.

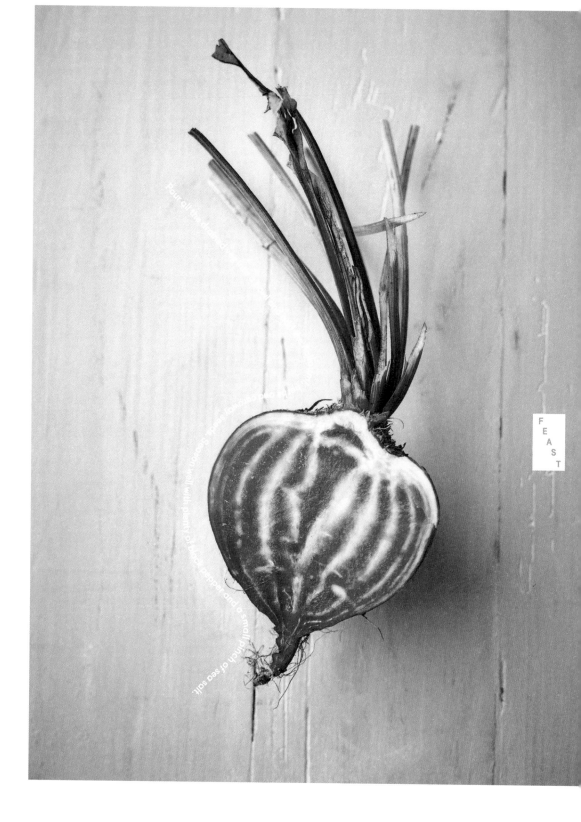

Pour all the drained fat... well with plenty of black pepper and a small pinch of sea salt.

Roasted cauliflower and butter bean salad with orange and olives

The addition of beans to the salad makes it a filling, nutritious main course that needs nothing by way of accompaniment. However, it goes brilliantly with a fillet of pan-fried white fish, such as sea bass or red mullet – in which case, it will definitely be enough for four.

Because you need to open a tin of beans for this and use a whole cauliflower and a whole orange, it's not really worth making a smaller amount. Just make it all and eat it cold the next day. It keeps really well.

**Serves 4 as a side dish,
or 2 as a main**
—

1 medium head cauliflower,
  cut into florets
  (about 400g)

2 tbsp extra-virgin olive oil

1 x 210g tin butter beans,
  drained and rinsed well

¼ red onion, very finely sliced

2 garlic cloves, crushed
  or very finely chopped

3 tbsp olive oil

2 tbsp sherry vinegar

1 tsp finely chopped
  rosemary

1 blood orange (or
  regular orange)

a few pitted black
  olives, halved

a small handful of flat-leaf
  parsley, very roughly
  chopped

flaked sea salt and freshly
  ground black pepper

Preheat the oven to 230°C/450°F/Gas mark 8. In a roasting tin, toss the cauliflower florets with the extra-virgin olive oil and a big pinch of salt. Roast for about 20 minutes, until the cauliflower is starting to char.

Meanwhile, combine the beans, onion, garlic, olive oil, sherry vinegar and rosemary in a large serving bowl.

Next, segment the orange. Using a sharp knife, top and tail the orange. Run your knife from the top to the bottom of the orange, removing a strip of skin and pith, following the curve of the fruit. Repeat all the way round – you'll probably have to repeat this 8–10 times to work your way around the whole orange. Now, holding it over a bowl, cut the segments out by cutting down either side of each membrane. You should end up with totally 'naked' segments without any pith or membrane. Once every segment is removed, squeeze the remaining core over the bowl to get all the juice out.

When the cauliflower is done, add to the bowl while still warm and mix with the beans, orange segments and dressing. Allow to cool to room temperature, then garnish with olives and parsley, season well, then serve.

Lentil and coconut dhal with spinach, toasted seeds, sprouts and tahini

Unlike your bog-standard dhal, this is an altogether more indulgent affair. The coconut milk makes it creamy and nutty, and it's still absolutely full of goodness. The toppings are optional, but together they really transform this dish into something pretty special.

This makes loads, so cook the whole batch and freeze the extra.

You can also add more stock and serve it as a soup. By all means use a shop-bought garam masala blend if you can't be bothered making your own.

Serves 4

2 tbsp olive oil, coconut oil or ghee

1 large onion, finely chopped

5cm piece of root ginger, peeled and finely grated

1 large garlic clove, finely chopped

1 tbsp garam masala (see right)

1 tsp dried chilli flakes

2 tsp nigella seeds

500g red lentils

1 litre vegetable stock (be ready to add more if you need to)

1 x 400ml tin coconut milk

50g baby spinach, roughly chopped

flaked sea salt and freshly ground black pepper

For the garam masala (optional)

1 tsp coriander seeds

1 tsp cumin seeds

1 cinnamon stick

2 cloves

¼ tsp black peppercorns

2 cardamom pods, crushed

1 star anise

1 bay leaf

To serve

4 tsp tahini

2 tsp Pear Café Seed Blend (see page 227)

4 tsp mixed sprouts

a few sprigs of coriander

If you're making the garam masala, dry toast all the spices in a small pan over a low heat until they start to release their aromas. Transfer to a spice grinder or mortar and pestle, and then grind to a fine powder. Set aside.

For the dhal, heat the oil in a pan and soften the onion, ginger and garlic over a medium-low heat for 10 minutes, until soft but not coloured. Add the dry spices, ginger, garlic and lentils, stirring thoroughly so that the lentils are coated in the oil and spices.

Pour in the stock and cook over a medium heat for about 30 minutes, until the lentils are tender. Add the coconut milk, remove from the heat and use a stick blender to blitz.

Place the pan back over a medium heat and stir through the spinach, until wilted. Taste for seasoning. Serve in bowls topped with the tahini, seeds, sprouts and coriander.

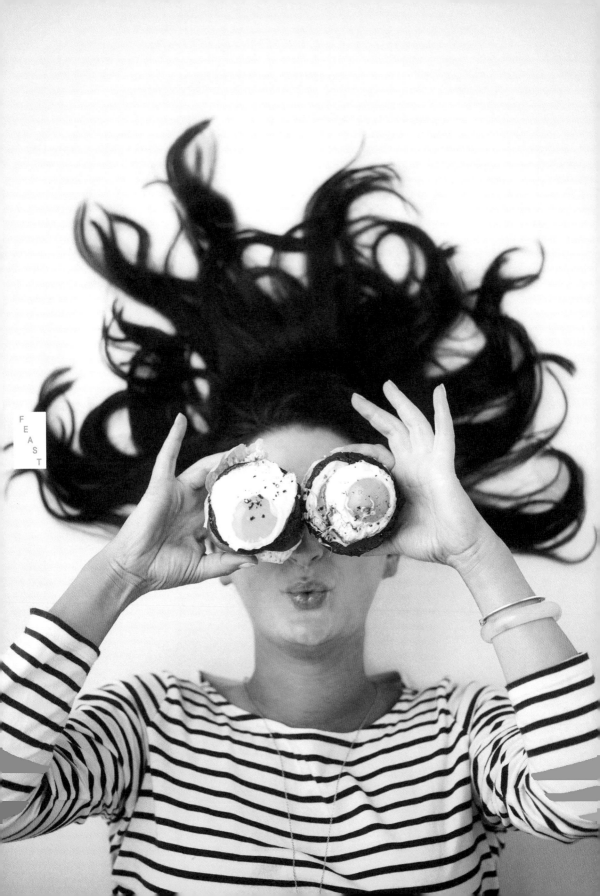

FEAST

Beetroot burgers

You can vary the herb and spice combo in these burgers. Try caraway with parsley or cumin with coriander. Think about other flavours that go well with beetroot – thyme, horseradish, goat's cheese, feta, dill and walnuts – and add them, too. These are best served with the Smoky Sweet Potato Wedges on page 145.

If you own a food processor, this is really quick and easy. You can do it by hand and grate the beetroot into the mixing bowl, but I recommend you wear rubber gloves.

Serves 4
—
4 x best-quality burger buns

For the burgers
1 x 400g tin chickpeas, drained and rinsed

2 tbsp olive oil, plus extra for frying

1 tsp toasted caraway or cumin seeds

approximately 2 tbsp toasted breadcrumbs

a small handful of finely chopped flat-leaf parsley or coriander (include the stalks)

150g raw beetroot

1½ tbsp flour

flaked sea salt and freshly ground black pepper

To serve (any combo of the following)
smoky avocado and chipotle mayo (see variation overleaf)

little gem lettuce

sliced tomato

gherkins, cut lengthways into 3mm slices

red onion, very finely sliced

China rose radish sprouts

Impatient Rainbow Pickles (see page 225)

fried egg

cheese (any you like)

Blitz all the ingredients for the burger, apart from the beetroot, flour and seasoning, in a food processor with the main chopping blade. Switch to a grating blade and grate the beetroot on top. Tip into a large bowl.

Shape the mixture into four even burgers. Combine the flour, salt and pepper in a shallow bowl. Dust the burgers with the seasoned flour.

Pour enough oil into a frying pan for shallow frying and place over a medium heat. Add the burgers and fry for 6–8 minutes, until browned. Flip over and brown on the other side. Check that the burgers are hot in the middle by inserting the tip of a sharp knife into the centre for a few seconds and then pulling it out: if the blade feels cold, cook the burgers for longer. If the outside browns too quickly, turn the heat right down.

Serve with your choice of toppings.

F
E
A
S
T

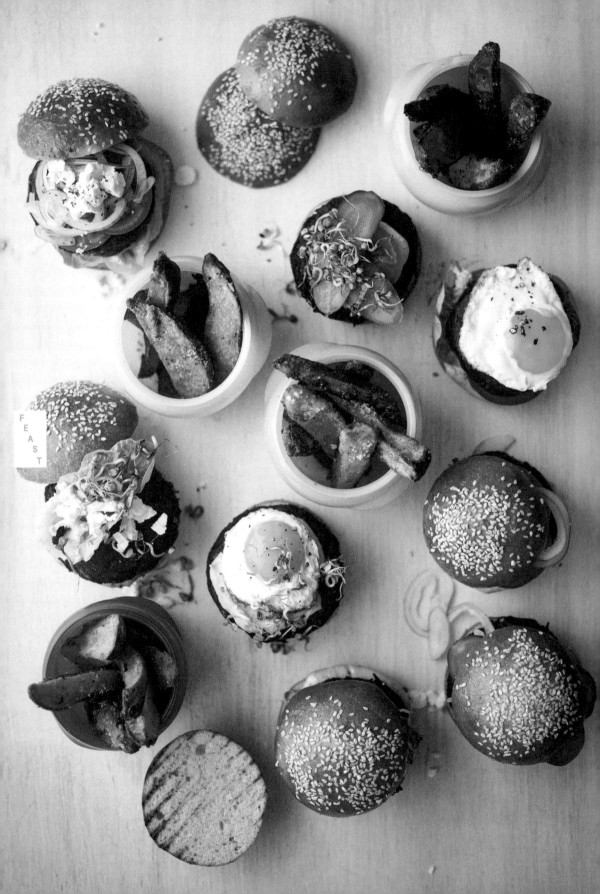

Smoky sweet potato wedges with tarragon and avocado mayo

Can I please just call this chips and béarnaise for hippies? 'Cos that's basically what it is.

This combo always makes me smile, because I only have to say the words 'chips and béarnaise' to my mate Dan and his eyes will roll back in his head, his tongue lolls out and you can't get proper sense out of him for a good few minutes until he comes round again from his little daydream. Steak, chips and béarnaise is his favourite thing of all time and the pure joy it brings him is totally understandable.

Serve these with any burger you like (or try them with the Beetroot Burgers on page 143), or eat them as a snack.

Serves 2

For the sweet potato wedges

300g sweet potato, cut into slim wedges

1 tbsp cornflour

2 tbsp olive oil

1 tsp sweet smoked paprika

1 tsp dried herbes de Provence

For the tarragon and avocado mayo

¼ avocado, destoned and roughly chopped

50g good-quality mayonnaise

1 garlic clove, roughly chopped

1 tbsp roughly chopped tarragon

flaked salt and freshly ground black pepper

Soak the sweet potato wedges in a large bowl of water for 1 hour.

Preheat the oven to 180°C/350°F/Gas mark 4.

Drain the wedges well. Put the cornflour into a large freezer bag and tip the wedges in. Trap air inside the bag and hold the top closed. Shake well to lightly dust the wedges with cornflour.

Mix the oil with the paprika and the dried herbs in a large bowl.

Pick the wedges out of the bag, one by one, shaking off the excess cornflour as you go, and add them to the bowl. Toss in the flavoured oil.

Spread out on a baking tray and, as best you can, stand them up on their 'skin' edges; this will make them extra crispy. Bake for 40 minutes until the edges start to char.

Meanwhile, make the tarragon and avocado mayo, by blitzing all the ingredients in a food processor until totally smooth. Season to taste.

Serve immediately with the avocado mayo. Like biscuits, these wedges will crisp up even more as they cool.

Note: You can change up the avocado mayo by replacing the tarragon with ½ teaspoon chipotle flakes. This smoky version goes really well with the Beetroot Burgers on page 143.

Marinated tofu
with
greens and brown rice

This is a dish I make over and over again at home. I absolutely love it and it's full of goodness. You can use any green veg and any rice or noodles you like. Big fat udon noodles are great, but my favourite is brown rice. It's one of those dishes you want to eat right now, as soon as you start thinking about it, and thankfully it doesn't take long to make. You could mix up the marinade in the morning and stick the tofu in, then as soon as you get home from work it can all be cooked and on the table in half an hour or less, depending on what rice or noodles you're serving with it. Use any seasonal green vegetables you have to hand – I've used a mixture of pak choi, tatsoi, choi sum and tenderstem broccoli and they work perfectly.

Serves 2

—

1 x 300g packet firm tofu, plain or smoked

200g seasonal green veg of choice

100g freshly cooked brown rice or noodles

3 tsp vegetable oil

For the tofu marinade

1 tbsp dark soy sauce

1 tbsp chilli and garlic sauce (available from Asian supermarkets)

½ tbsp sesame oil

For the garnish (any combination of the following, or all)

fresh coriander

6-minute egg (see page 16), halved

red chilli, finely sliced

spring onion, finely sliced

toasted sesame seeds

furikake (Japanese rice seasoning)

Take the tofu out of the packet and cut it into five or six slices. Lay the slices on one half of a doubled-over (clean and dry) tea towel and wrap the other side over, patting firmly to dry. Be very careful not to break the slices. Don't worry about getting it bone dry – you just want to dry it as much as you can.

Mix the marinade ingredients in a wide, shallow dish that will fit all the tofu slices.

Lay the tofu slices in the dish and gently toss them over so that they're evenly coated with the marinade. Allow to marinate for a while. An hour would be ideal, but even 10 minutes is fine. You can cook your rice now.

Prep the green veg. Soft leafy things like pak choi just need to have the leaves separated. Hardier greens like broccoli will need to be trimmed and cut into bite-sized pieces. Prep your garnishes – pick some nice coriander leaves. Get your finely sliced chilli and spring onion ready. Toast your sesame seeds. Get out your furikake. Say 'furry car key' out loud and laugh.

Heat the vegetable oil in a large frying pan or wok until hot. Fish the slices of tofu out of the dish and shake off any excess marinade. Carefully lay them in the pan. It's going to spit like mad, so don't wear white. Actually, wear an apron. And have a lid to hand to cover the pan if it starts going crazy.

Don't move the slices. Leave them alone for at least 4–5 minutes to get a nice crust before carefully flipping them over and frying the other side. When they're all brown on both sides, remove to a plate, cover loosely with foil and keep warm.

Slosh a bit of boiling water from the kettle into the pan. (This will act to deglaze the pan and create some steam to cook the veg.) Add the seasonal green veg to the pan along with the remaining marinade. Stir-fry for 2–3 minutes, over a medium–high heat, until all the veg is cooked but still crunchy.

Put your freshly cooked rice in a nice bowl and place the veg on top. Add the tofu and the garnishes. Take some soy sauce and sriracha to the table if you like.

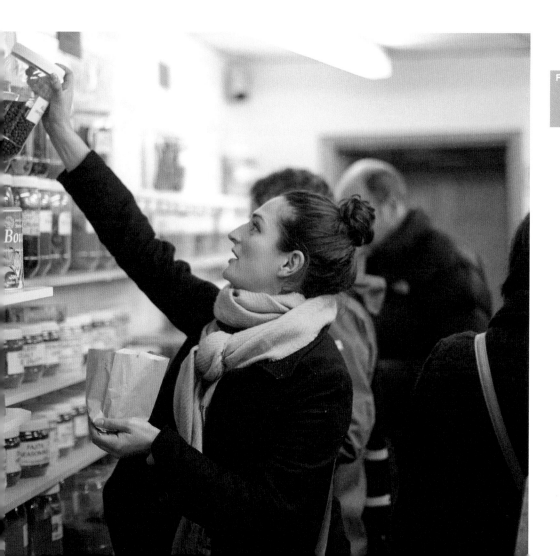

Cornershop stew

We started making this at the café and called it cornershop stew because everything we needed for it could be bought at any corner shop at any time of the day (and late into the night) and all year round. Oh, the joys of living and working in a city centre! It's a quick supper, using storecupboard ingredients that can also be blitzed up into a soup. Just add some more vegetable stock and use a stick blender to semi-blitz it.

It also happens to be both vegan and gluten free.

If you're serving it as a stew, I recommend serving it with some buttery kale and a big spoonful of Pico de Gallo (see page 235) on the side.

Serves 2
—

1 tbsp olive oil

1 medium onion, finely diced

50g Pear Café Seed
    Blend (see page 227)

1 heaped tbsp roughly
    chopped pickled
    jalapeños

2 tomatoes, roughly chopped

1 tsp vegetable bouillon
    powder

1 x 400g tin butter beans,
    drained and rinsed well

flaked sea salt and freshly
    ground black pepper

a handful of coriander,
    roughly chopped,
    to serve

Heat the olive oil in a pan and soften the onion, over a medium-low heat, covered, for 10 minutes until translucent. Stir in the seeds, jalapeños, tomatoes, bouillon powder, 150ml boiling water and the beans. Taste for seasoning and cook for 10 minutes. Serve, topped with the fresh coriander.

Done. Easy, eh?

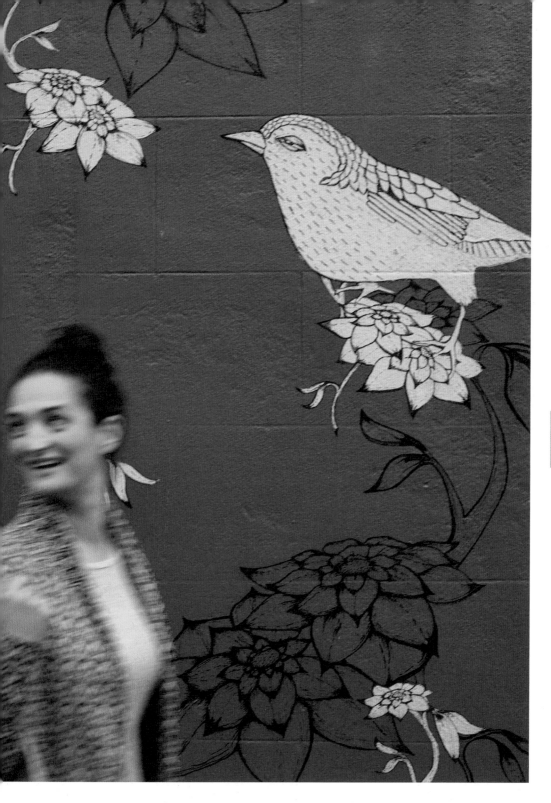

FEAST

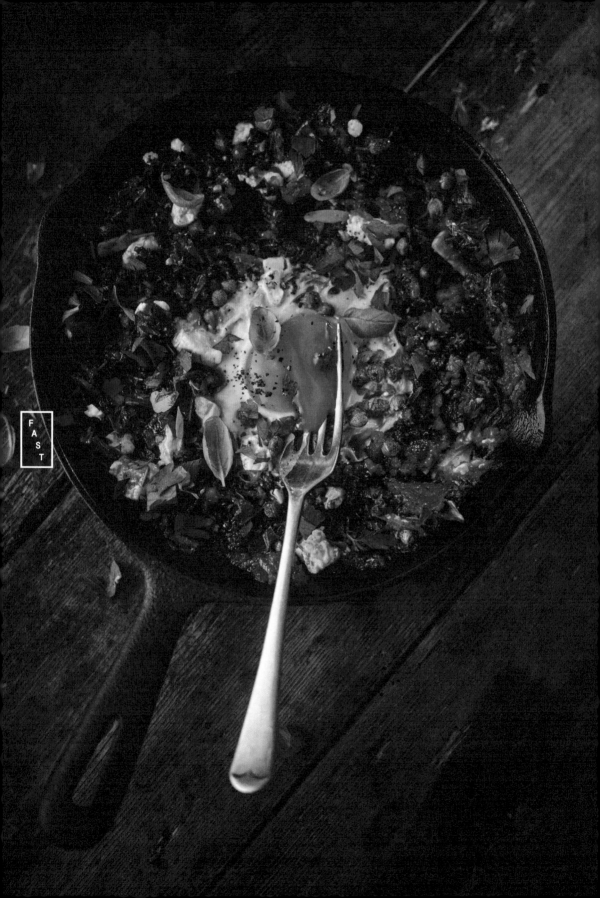

Eggs in purgatory with feta, kale and capers

217 kcal
per portion

Eggs in purgatory is very similar to the Israeli dish shakshuka. The bubbling hot chilli and tomato sauce that you slip the eggs into gives it its name.

This is a great dish for any time of day. On a feast day I love it for brunch, but it makes a great fast-day dinner, too. I've added feta, kale and capers to make it more substantial and nutritious yet low in calories. Keep the ingredients just as they are below on a fast day. On a feast day, you've got a few options: you can serve this with bread, add an extra egg, or simply be liberal with the feta and olive oil.

Serves 1

¼ tsp extra-virgin olive oil

1 garlic clove

3g red chilli, finely chopped

30g kale, finely chopped

100g tomato passata

150g tinned chopped tomatoes

1 egg

2 tsp capers, rinsed and drained

20g feta

1 tbsp chopped flat-leaf parsley

a few small basil leaves

flaked sea salt

Heat the oil in a small frying pan and cook the garlic and chilli over a medium heat for 2 minutes. Add the finely chopped kale and let it wilt for 5 minutes.

Add the passata, tinned tomatoes and a good pinch of salt. Let it come to the boil, then make a space in the centre of the tomatoes. Crack in the egg and sprinkle the capers and feta over the top.

Cover loosely with a lid or foil, and cook for about 5 minutes, just until the white of the egg is set.

Remove from the heat and sprinkle with parsley and basil.

Eat straight out of the pan.

F
A
S
T

Open lasagne

315 kcal
per portion

Lasagne on a fast day? Surely not? Well, okay, this is not the lasagne you might be dreaming of, with oozing layers of sauce and cheese. However, it's a clever way of getting a bit of delicious pasta into a fast day but balancing it with low-calorie vegetables, and it means you can satisfy your urge for a bit of lasagne action.

It isn't baked – you're basically making fresh pasta and a chunky sauce and layering it up.

Serves 1

1½ sheets fresh lasagne

2g Parmesan

For the roast vegetables

50g cherry tomatoes, halved

130g cooked beetroot, chopped into rough wedges

80g chestnut mushrooms, halved and larger ones quartered

50g red or yellow peppers, deseeded and roughly chopped

20g shallot, thinly sliced

¼ tsp extra-virgin olive oil

¼ tsp Turkish chilli flakes

flaked sea salt and freshly ground black pepper

For the sauce

200g tinned chopped tomatoes

2 anchovy fillets

a few basil leaves, plus extra to serve

Preheat the oven to 200°C/400°F/Gas mark 6.

Put the cherry tomatoes, beetroot, mushrooms, peppers and shallot in a roasting dish lined with greaseproof paper. Drizzle with the oil and season with salt and pepper. Sprinkle with the chilli flakes and roast in the oven for approximately 30 minutes, or until the vegetables are starting to char, are tender but still *al dente*.

Meanwhile, tip the tinned tomatoes into a small saucepan, season well, and then add the anchovy fillets and the basil leaves. Cook over a medium heat for about 15 minutes, until the anchovies have dissolved and the sauce has thickened and reduced.

When the roast veg are done, tip them into the pan and put a lid on. Keep warm over a very low heat while you cook the pasta sheets.

Boil the kettle and fill a medium-sized pan with the boiling water. Salt well.

Cut the whole sheet of fresh pasta in half – you're using three squares per person. (I tend to buy a packet, cut all the sheets in half and freeze them in sets of three squares, wrapped in cling film. You can then cook the sheets from frozen.)

Slip the pasta sheets into the boiling water and cook for 3–4 minutes until they're tender. Drain.

Put a quarter of the vegetable and sauce mixture in the middle of a warmed plate. Lay a sheet of pasta on top. Repeat the layering until all the sauce and pasta is used up, finishing with sauce on the top.

Shave or grate the Parmesan over the top and finish with a few extra basil leaves.

Serve with a big green salad.

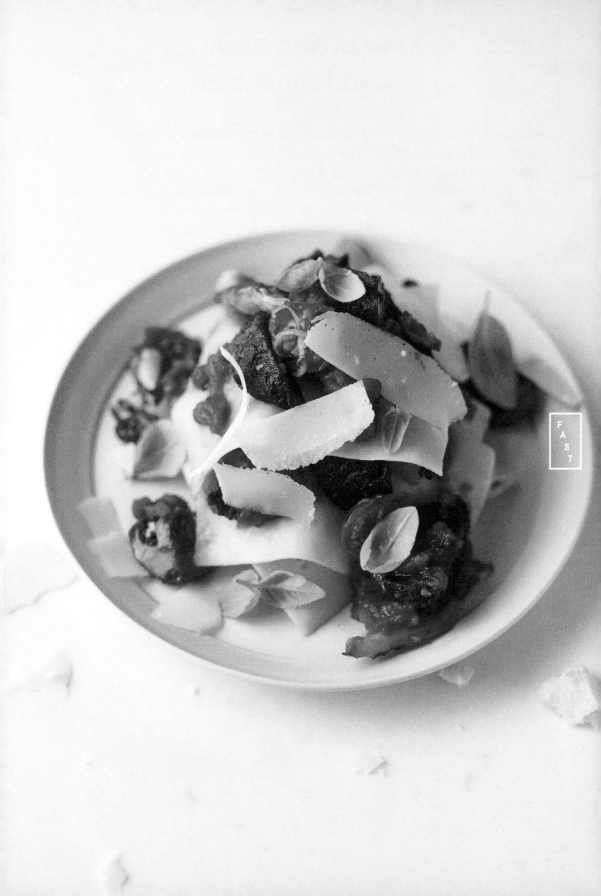

King prawn, celeriac and fennel stew

Fennel and prawns both feature regularly in my fast-day cooking. I most often use fennel raw, shredded into salads, where its crunch, strong flavour and mega-low calorie count all make it very welcome. When you cook fennel its flavour transforms and becomes very sweet and aromatic, and it works really well in tomato-based stews such as this. Here, a whole troop of low-calorie hero ingredients come together to create a dish that doesn't taste like a diet dish at all. On a feast day I'd finish it with a slick of peppery top-quality olive oil on the top, but even without that, it's still delicious. Swap pea shoots for watercress or rocket if you can't find them. The fresh, crunchy green on top really contrasts well with the hot stew.

Serves 1
—

¼ tsp extra-virgin olive oil

125g fennel, cut into wedges, fronds reserved

90g celeriac, peeled and cut into 2.5cm cubes

1 garlic clove, thinly sliced

1 tsp paprika

225g chopped tinned tomatoes

5g vegetable bouillon powder

70g cooked king prawns

10g pea shoots

flaked sea salt and freshly ground black pepper

Heat the oil in a medium-sized saucepan and cook the fennel and celeriac over a medium heat for 10 minutes, until softened. Add the garlic and paprika and season. Stir.

Add the tomatoes, bouillon powder and 125ml boiling water, or just enough to cover the celeriac. Cook for about 15 minutes, until the celeriac is totally tender.

Add the prawns and stir to heat through. Check and adjust the seasoning.

Serve in a bowl, garnished with the fennel fronds and pea shoots.

F
A
S
T

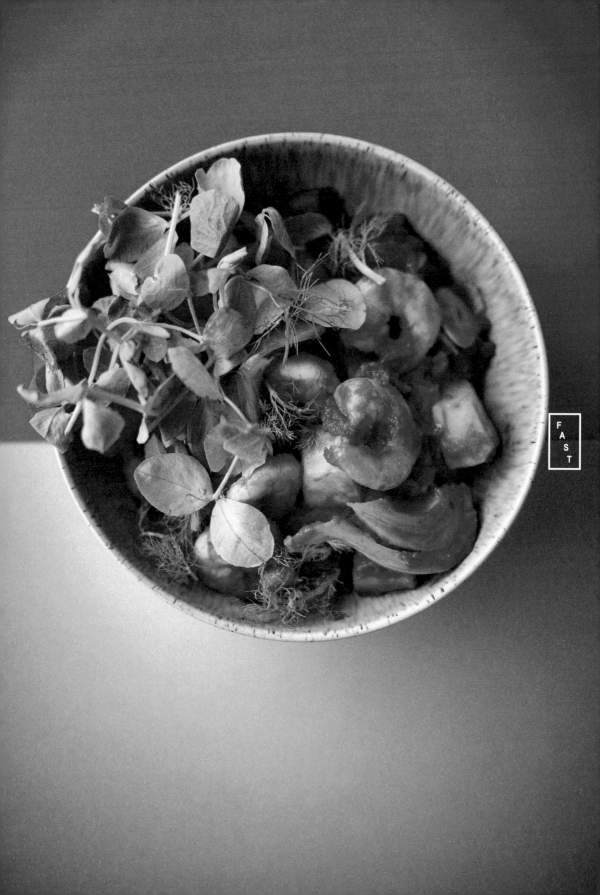

Kedgeree-ish

If you buy a packet of smoked haddock from the supermarket, portion it up and freeze it, well labelled, on the day you purchase. When I say labelled, I mean write the title, date and how many calories that portion is. If you can buy just the quantity you need from your fishmonger, even better.

You're using frozen peas and potentially frozen cauliflower rice that you've pre-prepared. If there is a portion of frozen haddock in the freezer too, you need to buy very little that's fresh.

Serves 1

—

1 egg

125g undyed smoked haddock fillet

1 bay leaf

100g raw cauliflower rice (see page 16)

20g frozen peas

1 teaspoon extra-virgin olive oil

25g red onion

2g curry powder

2.5ml soured cream

1 tbsp chopped flat-leaf parsley

½ tsp lemon juice

2g pea shoots

flaked sea salt and freshly ground black pepper

F
A
S
T

Cook the egg according to the 6-minute egg method (see page 16). When cool, slice into quarters and set aside.

Put the fish into a small pan and add the bay leaf. Cover with boiling water, bring back to the boil, put the lid on and remove from the heat. Leave to sit for 10 minutes. Drain well, reserving the cooking liquor.

Put the cauliflower rice into a medium-sized pan and pour over the reserved cooking liquor. Bring to the boil over a medium heat and simmer for 1 minute, just to heat through, then drain well. Set aside.

Cook the peas according to the packet instructions and drain well. Set aside.

Heat the oil in a pan and cook the onion over a medium-low heat for 10 minutes, until softened. Add the curry powder, stir, and cook for 3 minutes. Tip in the cauliflower rice, peas, soured cream and parsley and season to taste.

Flake the fish into the pan. Gently stir in the lemon juice and cook for a further 2 minutes. Place the egg quarters on the top, cover with the lid and heat through for about 2 minutes, until the egg is warmed.

Serve, topped with pea shoots.

Prawns, chickpeas
and
spring greens

194 kcal
per portion

Spring greens are cheap and plentiful in spring (surprise, surprise) and are very low in calories but with enough bite that they feel more substantial than something like spinach when cooked. Kale offers a good alternative when you can't get them.

Make this whole recipe and freeze one portion for another day or give a portion to a non-faster. It's a fast-day recipe that really doesn't taste like one.

Serves 4

—

1 tsp extra-virgin olive oil

2 garlic cloves, finely sliced

15cm twig rosemary

1 bay leaf

90g carrots, finely diced

40g celery, finely diced

30g red onion, finely diced

large pinch of flaked sea salt

1 x 400g tin cherry tomatoes

1 x 400g tin chickpeas, drained and rinsed well

5g vegetable bouillon powder, dissolved in 300ml boiling water

60g spring greens, cut into 1–2cm ribbons

140g cooked king prawns

1 tbsp chopped flat-leaf parsley

1 tsp finely grated lemon zest

Heat the oil in a large pan and add the garlic, rosemary twig, bay leaf, carrots, celery and onion. Add a large pinch of salt and stir well. Cover and cook the vegetables, stirring often, over a medium-low heat for about 10 minutes.

Add the tomatoes, chickpeas and stock and bring to the boil. Reduce the heat and simmer for 15 minutes.

Add the greens and cook for 10 more minutes. Add the prawns and cook for 2–3 minutes until they are pink but not tough.

Plate up and sprinkle with parsley and lemon zest.

F
A
S
T

Winter greens fritter with smoked trout and chrain

This is a real cracker – quick, filling, delicious, adaptable. It's got a great variety of textures and is also a perfect feast-day brunch dish or the basis of a light lunch or supper. On a feast day, I'd add an extra egg to the mix, use both olive oil and butter to fry it in (to get a really great crust on the fritter) and perhaps add some sliced cooked new potatoes in, too, which would make it more of a frittata.

I grew up eating chrain (pronounced as if you're trying to clear your throat and say Rhine at the same time – a real skill), which is a beetroot and horseradish relish. Some brands are hotter than others, but I am yet to find a brand that I don't like. You can buy it in Kosher delis or Polish shops, where you'll see it labelled as ćwikła z chrzanem. It's cheap and, as I recently discovered, low in calories. It's a bright pinky-red, punchy and looks and tastes great alongside the smoked trout. Once you've opened the jar, I bet you find loads of ways to use it.

If you can't get hold of the smoked trout fillets, you could substitute poached or smoked salmon. As with all amendments and substitutions, make sure you carefully recalculate the correct calorie count.

F
A
S
T

Serves 1

—

75g cabbage, greens
or kale, roughly chopped

1 tsp olive oil

1 free-range medium egg,
separated

10g rocket

45g smoked trout, flaked

5g spring onion, sliced

15g chrain

flaked sea salt and freshly
ground black pepper

Rinse the greens and shake them nearly dry. Heat ½ teaspoon olive oil (very carefully measured) in a small (15–20cm) non-stick frying pan over a medium heat, add the damp greens, cover and let them wilt in their own steam after 1–2 minutes. Drain off any excess liquid and season well.

Put the greens in a bowl and set aside. Wipe the pan clean with kitchen paper.

Whisk the egg white in a very clean, grease-free bowl until holding firm peaks. Break the yolk and fold it into the whites. Add to the greens.

Put the remaining ½ teaspoon olive oil in the pan and tip in the greens mixture. Use a spoon to evenly distribute the greens in the pan and right up to the edges. Leave to set for about 4 minutes, and then flip to brown both sides.

Slide the fritter onto a plate and top with the rocket, add the flaked smoked trout, then top with the spring onion and the chrain.

Serve.

Lemon sole with celeriac colcannon and kale

186 kcal per portion

This is one of my recipes that Gizzi Erskine featured in her *Sunday Times Magazine* column in January 2015. I'd been doing the 5:2 for a long time already at that point, so when she asked me for some really cracking fast-day recipes, I had plenty to choose from. I knew this one definitely had to be included because when I'd first made it and posted a picture on Instagram, Marina O'Loughlin, the *Guardian*'s restaurant critic, had commented, 'Bloody hell. That's an amazing one. *impressed*'. She's not one to hand out praise lightly, so I put a big star by this recipe in my notebook.

Serves 1

110g peeled celeriac, chopped

60ml semi-skimmed milk

1 garlic clove, crushed

25g kale, roughly chopped

80g lemon sole

3g plain flour

¼ tsp extra-virgin olive oil

5g unsalted butter

flaked sea salt and freshly ground black pepper

Put the celeriac into a small pan and add the milk and crushed garlic. Add just enough water to top up and cover the celeriac. Simmer gently for about 15 minutes, until tender. Drain the celeriac, reserving the liquid, and mash. Season well. Add a few splashes of the liquid into the mash if it seems too dry.

Bring a pan of water to the boil, add the kale and blanch for 5 minutes. Drain and allow to cool enough to handle. Chop up and add the kale to the celeriac mash. Keep warm.

Pat the fish nearly dry with kitchen paper and cut in half lengthways, so you have two small fillets.

Dust a small plate with the flour and season well. Press the fish into the flour and turn so all the sides are lightly covered.

Put the oil and the butter into a frying pan and heat over a medium heat, until the butter is melted. Fry the fish for 2 minutes on each side, until crisp and golden.

To serve, pile the colcannon onto the middle of a plate and drape the fish fillets across the top.

FAST

Cajun prawns

These prawns are smoky and spicy and make a delicious dish when accompanied by the Celeriac 'grits' (see opposite). They also work well cold, so make the whole batch and save half for lunch the next day. Serve them with chilled cauliflower rice or a slaw. The parsley and lemon really lift the whole dish — don't leave them out either.

The spice mix could be made up in advance in larger quantities and kept in a jar to be used whenever you need it. It's the same blend used in the Jambalaya-ish recipe (page 162) and can also be used in loads of other ways — sprinkled over freshly popped popcorn; mixed with oil, brushed over salmon and then grilled; or sprinkled over potato wedges before baking.

Serves 2

240g raw king prawns, peeled and deveined

1 tsp extra-virgin olive oil

40g red onion, very finely diced

1 garlic clove, crushed

pinch of flaked sea salt

1½ tsp lemon juice, plus wedges to serve

1 tbsp roughly chopped flat-leaf parsley

For the seasoning

½ tsp smoked paprika

½ tsp cayenne pepper

½ tsp dried oregano

½ tsp dried thyme

½ tsp dried chilli flakes

Mix all the seasoning ingredients in a small bowl.

Pat the prawns dry with kitchen paper and toss them in the spice mix. Set aside.

Heat the oil in a frying pan over a medium heat. Cook the onion and garlic, with a pinch of salt, gently for 5 minutes with the lid on, until softened. Remove the lid and add the prawns. Cook for about 5 minutes, over a medium heat, until they turn pink. Add the lemon juice and sauté for another 2 minutes.

Remove from the heat and sprinkle with parsley.

Serve on a bed of celeriac grits (see opposite) with a lemon wedge on the side.

Celeriac 'grits'

91 kcal
per portion

You can 'rice' celeriac the way you can 'rice' cauliflower. It's similarly low calorie and really cheap. Don't let a celeriac's rather ugly appearance put you off. Trim it and inside its knobbly exterior it is creamy white and has a deliciously nutty, mild celery flavour.

'Grits' are a southern American dish, very similar to polenta and likewise made with ground corn. You want to blitz your celeriac to a much finer crumb than when you're making cauliflower rice.

Serves 2

520g peeled celeriac
1 tsp olive oil
90g onions, diced
1 garlic clove, crushed
5g vegetable bouillon powder, dissolved in 500ml boiling water
flaked sea salt and freshly ground black pepper

Cut the celeriac into 2.5cm cubes and blitz in a food processor until you have a very fine texture, like grits. Set aside.

Heat the oil in a medium saucepan over a medium heat, add the onions, salt and pepper and cook until the onions begin to soften and brown.

Add the garlic, stock and celeriac and stir. Cover and cook over a low heat for 10 minutes, stirring regularly. Take off the lid and cook for a further 10–15 minutes until most of the liquid has evaporated. Serve.

FAST

Jambalaya-ish

Jambalaya is a Louisiana Creole dish and traditionally a carnivore's dream, with chicken, sausage and prawns elbow to elbow, and sometimes all sorts of other things like alligator and squirrel. There are a million different recipes out there. While in no way a 'traditional' Jambalaya (hence the -ish), my version uses the classic combo of onion, celery and green pepper, and the Creole spice blend of cayenne, paprika, oregano and thyme. I keep the prawns and use cauliflower rice to make a pescetarian, fast-day-friendly spin-off, which is still delicious.

Serves 1

—

1 tsp olive oil

30g red onion, finely chopped

30g celery, finely diced

30g green pepper, deseeded and finely diced

140g tomatoes

1 garlic clove, crushed

¼ tsp Cajun Spice Blend (see page 228)

1 bay leaf

80g raw cauliflower rice (see page 16)

70g cooked king prawns

10g spring onion, finely sliced

sea salt and freshly ground black pepper

F
A
S
T

Heat the oil in a frying pan over a medium heat. Add the onion, celery and pepper, and cook over a medium heat for 8–10 minutes.

Place the tomatoes in a bowl and pour over boiling water. Leave for 5 minutes and then rinse under cool running water. Make a cross at the base of each tomato and then slip off the skins. Roughly chop.

Add the garlic, Cajun spice blend and bay leaf to the pan and cook for 30 seconds, stirring. Stir in the tomatoes, including all their juices from the board, and cook for 5 minutes. Add the cauliflower rice, season well, add a little water and stir well, scraping up the bottom of the pan.

Stir in the prawns and cook for another 2 minutes to heat them through.

Plate up and garnish with the spring onion.

Steamed eggs

There are various steamed egg recipes all over Asia, from Korean geran chim to chawanmushi from Japan to Chinese 'steamed water eggs'.

They're all basically a smooth, set, savoury egg custard, seasoned and strewn with various toppings.

This recipe is fast-day friendly, but on a feast day simply relax and add whatever you like to the top, without having to weigh or measure anything. I think mushrooms in a sticky miso glaze would be amazing.

Serves 1

—

2 eggs

1 tsp miso paste

6 x (½ an eggshell) boiled then cooled water

¼ tbsp rice wine vinegar

For the topping

¼ tsp sesame oil

3g spring onion, finely sliced

1 tsp light soy sauce

Fill a small lidded saucepan with water, up to about 2.5cm deep. Bring to the boil.

Crack the eggs in a bowl and whisk together with the remaining ingredients. Strain through a fine sieve or tea strainer into a shallow heatproof dish. (I use a small Chinese-style teacup.) Pop/remove any bubbles.

Cover with cling film and carefully place the heatproof bowl in the pan of water. Cover with the lid and steam for about 15 minutes, until set.

Remove carefully and put to one side.

Heat the sesame oil in a small pan.

Very carefully (the steam will be hot, so don't burn your fingers) remove the cling film. Scatter with the spring onion and immediately pour the hot oil over. This will release the fragrance of the onion. Drizzle the soy sauce over the top and serve straight away.

F
A
S
T

How to Build a Buddha Bowl

Buddha bowls are basically big, hearty salads. They're built on a combination of grains and greens, then topped with all sorts of interchangeable things. They're filling, portable, don't wilt and go sad, and they are endlessly adaptable. There's no right or wrong way to create a Buddha bowl – you can make a simple one or get really creative.

Most nights, my dinner is a variation on this idea. I'm sure some would argue that you should be giving your full attention to the Buddha bowl, probably followed by a spot of meditation and yoga, but I find them to be excellent as TV dinners.

They are brilliant receptacles for leftovers and even if you have a tiny bit of something left, you can add it to the top.

Following these rough quantities ensures that you will get a good balance of fat, protein and carbs, but don't worry too much about getting quantities spot on. Just concentrate on getting as much veg as possible in there and treating the other elements as the (albeit important) support acts. If you're a meat eater, this is the perfect way to showcase a really excellent piece of top-quality meat. Eating less but better-quality meat is better for you and the planet. Try to stop seeing meat as the centre of your plate and instead treat it as they do in much of the world – as almost a garnish. The majority of the bowl will consist of cheap grains and veg, so spending a little extra on organic meat (or eggs or some fancy schmancy tofu) will be balanced out.

Pick at least one element from each section, making up at least half of the total with veg, a quarter of beans/pulses, and the rest from the remaining sections.

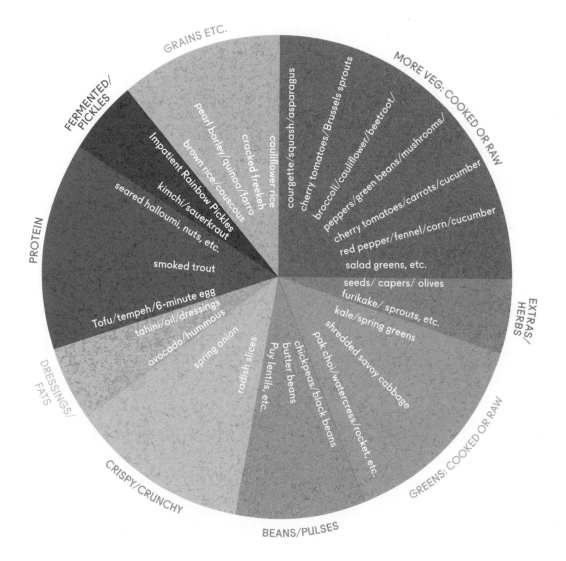

GRAINS ETC.

FERMENTED/
PICKLES

MORE VEG: COOKED OR RAW

asparagus/courgettes
Brussels sprouts/cherry tomatoes
/beetroot/cauliflower/broccoli
mushrooms/green beans/peppers
cucumber/carrots/cherry tomatoes
cucumber/corn/fennel/red pepper
salad greens, etc.
seeds/ capers/ olives
furikake/ sprouts, etc.

cauliflower rice
cracked freekeh
pearl barley/quinoa/farro
brown rice/couscous
Impatient Rainbow Pickles
kimchi/sauerkraut

PROTEIN

seared halloumi, nuts, etc.

smoked trout

EXTRAS/
HERBS

kale/spring greens
shredded savoy cabbage
pak choi/watercress/rocket, etc.

Tofu/tempeh/6-minute egg
tahini/oil/dressings
avocado/hummous
spring onion
radish slices
Puy lentils, etc.
butter beans
chickpeas/black beans

DRESSINGS/
FATS

CRISPY/CRUNCHY

GREENS: COOKED OR RAW

BEANS/PULSES

165 — Weeknight Dinners

Salmon rice bowl

Getting a really crisp skin on a piece of salmon makes it infinitely better. If you don't think you like fish skin, I guarantee it's flabby fish skin you don't like. Crispy, well-seasoned salmon skin is manna from heaven. The way it contrasts with the rich, soft fish flesh is incredible. Add the nuttiness of the brown rice, the crunch of the pickles and the lusciousness of the sour cream and avocado and you've got a winner winner, salmon dinner.

Serves 2

—

175g short-grain brown rice, freshly cooked

2 x 200g salmon steaks, skin on

olive oil

2 tbsp soured cream

2 heaped tbsp Impatient Rainbow Pickles (see page 225)

¼ ripe avocado

1 small bunch of coriander

2 tsp Pear Café Seed Blend (see page 227)

flaked sea salt and freshly ground black pepper

Cook the rice according to the instructions on p17. When the rice is 10 minutes from being done, start the salmon.

Pat your salmon steaks dry with kitchen paper, then rub all over with a little olive oil. Lay on a plate, skin side up, and season with salt and pepper.

Preheat your frying pan over a high heat. (At this point I'd turn the extractor fan on/open the windows, too.) Carefully lay the salmon in the pan, skin side down. Press down on the surface of the fish to make sure the skin is in full contact with the hot pan. Do not move the fish. Leave it still for at least 4 minutes, so that you get a good char on the skin. Watch carefully as the fish cooks and the bright pink flesh turns slowly opaque from the skin upwards. Once that 'cooked' line is halfway up, turn the heat off and, very carefully, using a palette knife, flip the salmon over. The residual heat of the pan cooks the fish.

Drain the rice and divide between two bowls. Lay the fish on top, skin side up, and add a spoonful of soured cream and pickles to each bowl. Slice the avocado and divide the slices between the bowls. Finish with a few coriander leaves and a sprinkling of toasted seeds.

Season the dish and serve.

Other nice things with seared salmon

4 tablespoons Coconut and Lime Dressing (see page 234), mixed with two big handfuls of cooked Puy lentils, topped with the seared salmon, fresh coriander and lime wedges.

Raw beetroot slaw made from shredded multi-coloured beets, dressed with a little olive oil, and mixed with lots of coriander, parsley, mint and fresh red chilli.

Cooked noodles dressed with the Tahini Noodle Dressing (see page 229) and serve with stir-fried broccoli with seared salmon on top. Add the Pear Café Seed Blend (page 227) and finely sliced spring onion.

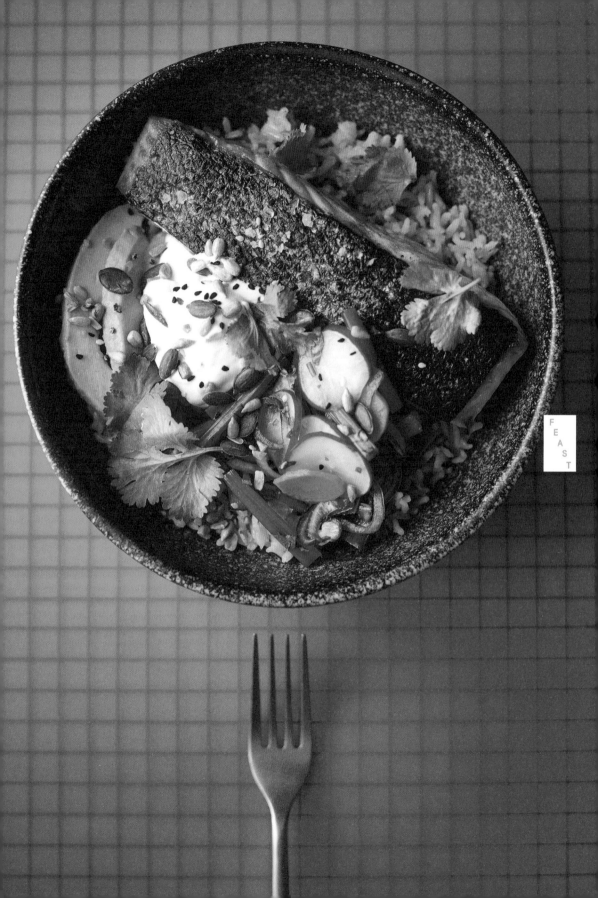

FEAST

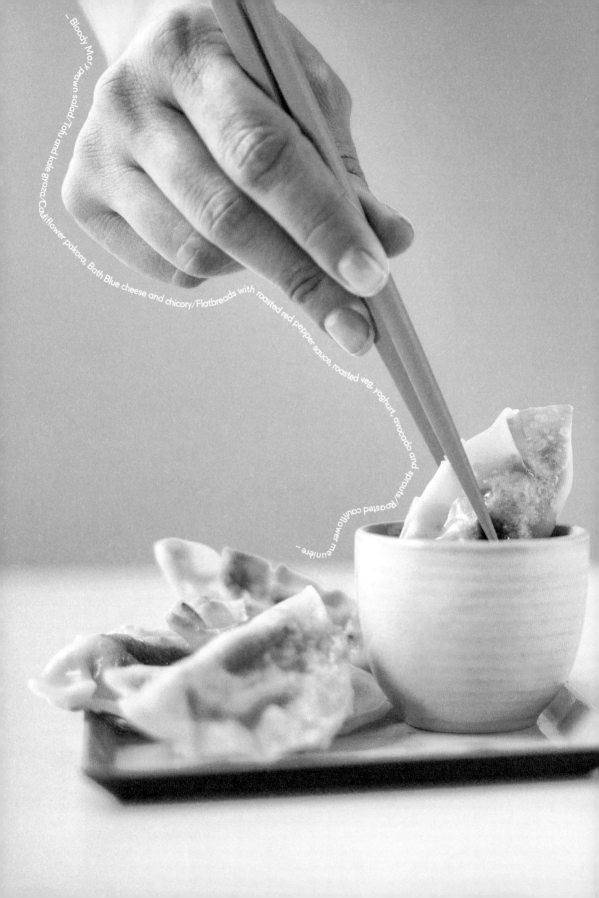

~ Bloody Mary prawn salad/Tofu and kale gyoza/Cauliflower pakora, Bath Blue cheese and chicory/Flatbreads with roasted red pepper sauce, roasted veg, yoghurt, avocado and sprouts/Roasted cauliflower meunière ~

Weekend Cooking
and
Entertaining

Flatbreads with roasted red pepper sauce, roasted veg, yoghurt, avocado and sprouts

These make the perfect Friday night dinner on the sofa — a kind of healthy mix between a taco and a pizza. It's not covered in loads of cheese and the flatbreads are piled up with veg so you'd be getting your weekend off to a healthy start. Serve with the Mexican Avocado Chopped Salad on page 63 and feel mega-virtuous for a few hours (even if the rest of the weekend is a drunken blur).

Serves 2

—

1 x quantity flatbreads (see page 137), or cheat and use 4 shop-bought flatbreads/pittas

1 x quantity roasted red pepper sauce (see page 229), or good-quality shop-bought red pepper pesto

1 ripe avocado, destoned and sliced

4 tbsp Greek yoghurt

4 tsp Wild Garlic Oil (see page 237), or pesto or plenty of chopped fresh herbs (optional)

small handful of alfalfa sprouts

small handful of radish sprouts

4 lime wedges

flaked sea salt and freshly ground black pepper

For the roast vegetables

1 sweet potato, cut into 2.5cm cubes

¼ medium cauliflower, broken into florets

2 tbsp olive oil or coconut oil

¼ tsp smoked paprika

¼ tsp Turkish chilli flakes

¼ tsp ground coriander

¼ tsp ground cumin

First, roast your vegetables. Preheat the oven to 220°C/430°F/Gas mark 7. In a large bowl, toss the sweet potato and cauliflower in the olive oil and spices and season with salt and pepper. Spread out evenly on a baking tray lined with baking parchment and roast for about 30 minutes, until the sweet potato is tender and the cauliflower has started to char at the edges.

While the veg is roasting, make your flatbreads as directed on page 137, if using homemade. If using shop-bought pittas, warm under the grill.

Spread 2 tablespoons roasted red pepper sauce on each flatbread.

Remove the roast veg from the oven and divide between the flatbreads, along with the avocado slices.

Top with the yoghurt, sprouts and wild garlic oil, then tuck a lime wedge on the side, season with salt and pepper, then serve.

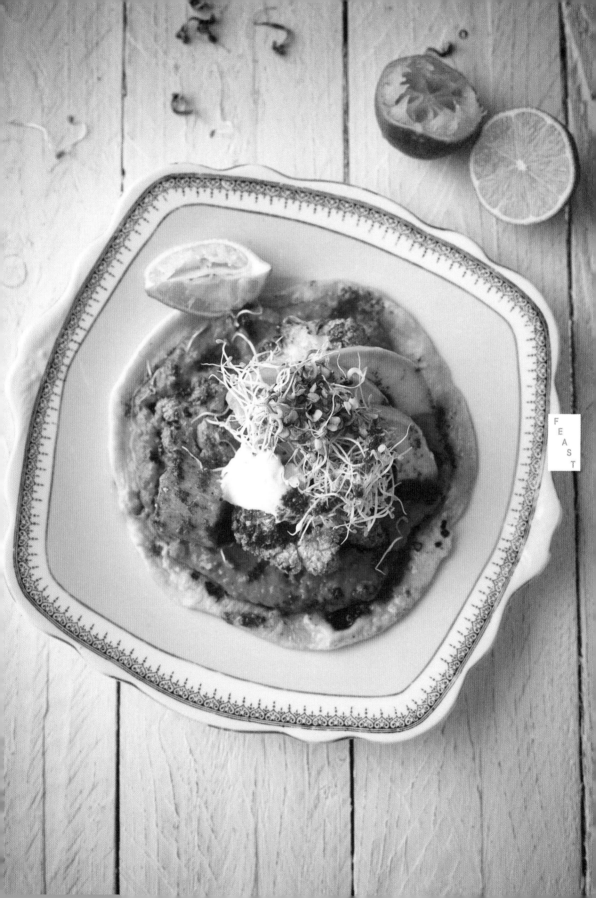

Tofu and kale gyoza

You can eat these Japanese-style dumplings on a fast day on two conditions: you make them and weigh out the fillings really carefully and you just use half a teaspoon of oil to fry five of them. That equals 166 kcal (including the dipping sauce), so obviously you can do more if you've got the calorie space.

I taught myself how to fold the gyoza from a YouTube Video. I suggest you do the same. It's impossible to describe in words – you need to watch someone do it. I made gyoza for the very first time, while trying to learn how to fold them, on a fast day. DO NOT follow my example on this one! Make them on a feast day and freeze. You can cook them from frozen and make a really speedy fast-day dinner. Please note, you must initially freeze them in a flat, single layer, on greaseproof paper and not touching. Once they are totally frozen, you can transfer them into a freezer bag and they won't all stick together.

I serve them on a feast day with the Ginger and Miso dressing (see page 222) with a swirl of hoisin sauce on top also to dip into and slices of avocado on the side. Lush.

FAST

Serves 4

30g spring onions, roughly chopped

¼ tbsp grated root ginger

1 garlic clove, crushed

30g kale leaves, roughly chopped

230g firm plain tofu, drained

50g water chestnuts, very finely chopped

1 tbsp light soy sauce

¼ tbsp rice vinegar

1 tsp sesame oil

20 wonton wrappers

vegetable oil, for frying

freshly ground black pepper

Make the dipping sauce first by combining all the ingredients in a small bowl and mixing well. Set to one side.

Blitz the spring onions, ginger and garlic in a food processor until the mixture is close to a rough paste. Add the kale and pulse-blend until everything is evenly combined. Add the tofu and pulse again until roughly incorporated. Add the water chestnuts, soy sauce, vinegar, sesame oil and a grinding of black pepper, and blend until you have the desired consistency. Occasionally use a spatula to scrape down the sides and incorporate everything evenly.

Fill a small bowl with water. Place about ½ tablespoon of tofu filling into the centre of one wonton wrapper. Use your finger to dab a little water around half of the wrapper's edge and fold over to form a half-moon shape; pinch the edges to seal. Repeat with the remaining filling and wrappers.

Once all the dumplings are prepared, heat a large pan over a medium heat. Once hot, add a little vegetable oil, just enough to coat the pan. Add the dumplings, in a single layer (they should start to sizzle when they hit the pan), and fry for 1–2 minutes, or until a golden crust starts to develop on the bottom. Flip and cook for another 1–2 minutes, so that a crust forms on the other side (at this stage, the gyoza will still appear mostly uncooked). Add

For the dipping sauce
60ml rice vinegar
60ml light soy sauce
pinch of dried chilli flakes
¼ garlic clove, crushed
½ tsp finely grated root ginger
¼ spring onion, finely sliced

a few tablespoons of water, cover the pan loosely and let the gyoza steam for 1 minute. When you remove the lid, the gyoza should look glossy and slightly translucent around the edges. If they're really sticking to the pan, add a little more water to help loosen them. Continue to cook the remaining gyoza this way. To serve, put five gyoza on each plate and have the dipping sauce on the side.

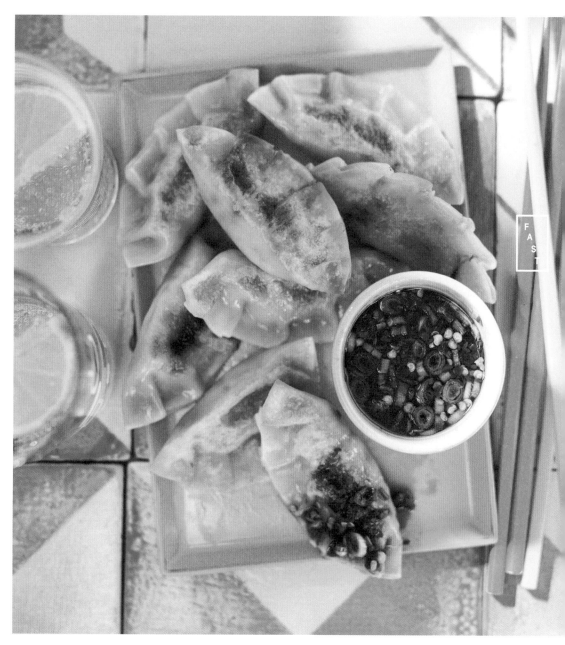

F
A
S
T

Cauliflower pakora, Bath Blue cheese and chicory

This was the veggie main course at the #salonxellypear pop-up I did with Nicholas Balfe from Brixton's Salon Restaurant. We cooked for over 70 people in Yurt Lush, the aptly named yurt in Bristol. Devised as part of a seven-course menu, but you can serve it as a main, in which case it will feed four.

I discovered Bath Blue cheese via one of my café babes, Jen. Her partner Joe makes it himself by hand. If that's not cool enough, they've also won numerous awards, including The World Champion trophy at the 2014 World Cheese Awards, the biggest in the industry. It really is the big cheese.

Serves 6, as a starter
—

For the cauliflower pakoras

150g chickpea flour

1 tsp sea salt

¼ tsp turmeric

¼ tsp ground coriander

¼ tsp chilli powder

¼ tsp garam masala

½ tsp bicarbonate of soda

1 tsp nigella seeds

Rapeseed oil, for deep-frying

500g cauliflower florets

flaked sea salt, for sprinkling

To serve

120g Bath blue cheese, or other creamy blue cheese of choice

16 red chicory leaves

rocket flowers (optional)

Wild garlic oil, for drizzling (see page 237)

6 heaped tbsp Brown Butter (see page 234), melted

Put the chickpea flour, salt, turmeric, coriander, chilli powder and garam masala in a large bowl and gradually whisk in 150ml water, until you have a thick, smooth batter. Leave to stand for 10 minutes.

When you're ready to serve, stir in the bicarbonate of soda and the nigella seeds.

Heat the oil in a large, deep frying pan until it reaches 180°C/350°F, or test if the oil is hot by dipping a tiny piece of cauliflower in the batter, shaking off the excess, and dropping it carefully in the oil. If it browns in 45 seconds, the oil is hot enough.

To cook the pakoras, dip the cauliflower florets in the batter, shaking off the excess as before. Gently drop a few pieces into the hot oil – don't drop from a height – but be careful not to splash hot oil on your hand. Fry a few pieces at a time so as not to overcrowd the pan. Deep-fry for about 8 minutes, or until the batter is puffed up and golden brown.

Remove from the oil with a slotted spoon and drain the pakoras on kitchen paper. Immediately sprinkle with flaked sea salt. They'll stay hot for ages, so don't worry too much about the first batch cooling down.

To serve, place a few pakoras on each serving plate and crumble the Bath Blue around them. Add a few red chicory leaves and rocket flowers. Finish with a drizzle of the herb oil and brown butter, then serve.

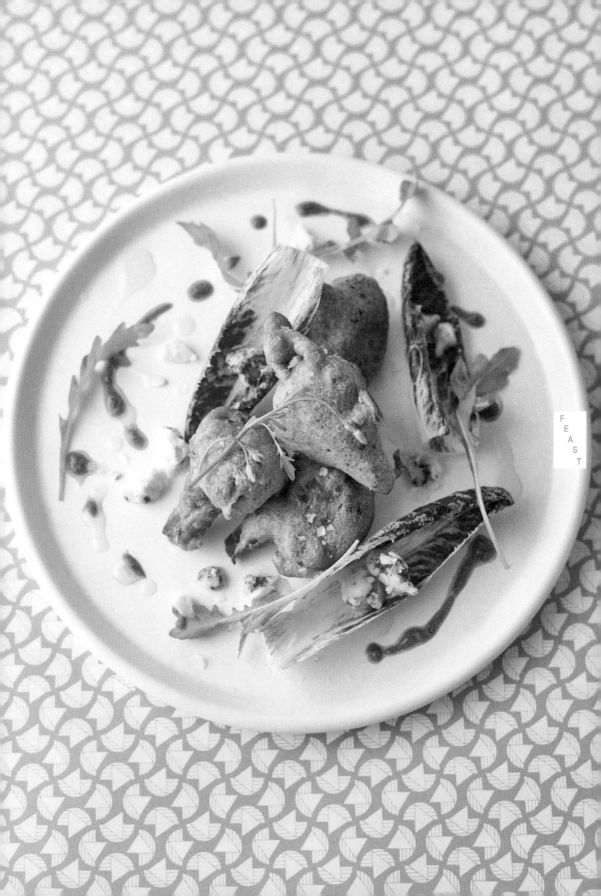

Friday night one-pot quinoa bowl with smoky roast tomatoes and avocado

This is simple and quick – you just chuck it all in one pot and leave it – but it feels like a real treat. It's perfect Friday night food, hence the name, when you want something special but are too tired to spend ages cooking. You can make a couple of the elements ahead of time: the tomatoes can be roasted and kept covered in the fridge; the tortilla chips can be stored in an airtight container. It will make the dish even quicker to throw together. If you're feeling really lazy and can't be fussed making the roast tomatoes and chips in advance, simply roughly chop some cherry tomatoes and buy some nachos.

Serves 4

For the smoky roast tomatoes

250g cherry tomatoes, halved

1 tsp Cajun Spice Blend
(see page 228)

1 tbsp olive oil

For the tortilla chips

1 tortilla wrap, cut into
8 triangles

olive oil spray

For the quinoa

1 tbsp olive oil

2 garlic cloves, finely chopped

1 tbsp roughly chopped
pickled jalapeños

1 x 400g tin black beans,
drained and rinsed

165g frozen sweetcorn,
or tinned sweetcorn

1 tsp vegetable bouillon
powder

180g quinoa, toasted

2 tsp Cajun Spice Blend
(see page 228)

sea salt and freshly ground
black pepper

To serve

100g feta, crumbled

1 ripe avocado, destoned
and sliced

4 lime wedges

1 small handful of chopped
coriander

4 tsp toasted pumpkin seeds

4 heaped tbsp Pico de Gallo
(see page 235), optional

Preheat the oven to 180°C/350°F/Gas mark 4.

To make the smoky roast tomatoes, combine all
the ingredients together in a bowl and toss well so
the tomatoes are coated all over in the spiced oil.
Tip the tomatoes into a roasting tray lined with baking
parchment and spread out evenly. Roast for 30 minutes,
or until the tomatoes are starting to char and collapse.
Remove from the oven and set aside.

About 15 minutes before the tomatoes are done, make
the tortilla chips. Spray the triangular pieces on both
sides in a light coating of olive oil. Arrange them
in a single layer on a baking tray and put them
in the oven for the final 10 or so minutes of the
tomatoes cooking time, until the chips are
golden. Remove and sprinkle with salt.

Next, make the quinoa. Heat the olive oil in
a large pan (that you have a lid for), add the
garlic and cook for 1 minute, until starting to
brown. Add the remaining ingredients for
the quinoa along with 250ml boiling water
and bring to the boil over high heat. Reduce
to low heat and simmer, covered, for
20 minutes until the quinoa is just tender.

Taste for seasoning and divide between
four bowls.

Top with the crumbled feta, avocado slices,
lime wedges, fresh coriander, tortilla chips,
pumpkin seeds and a spoonful each of pico
de gallo (if using).

Best served with cold beer.

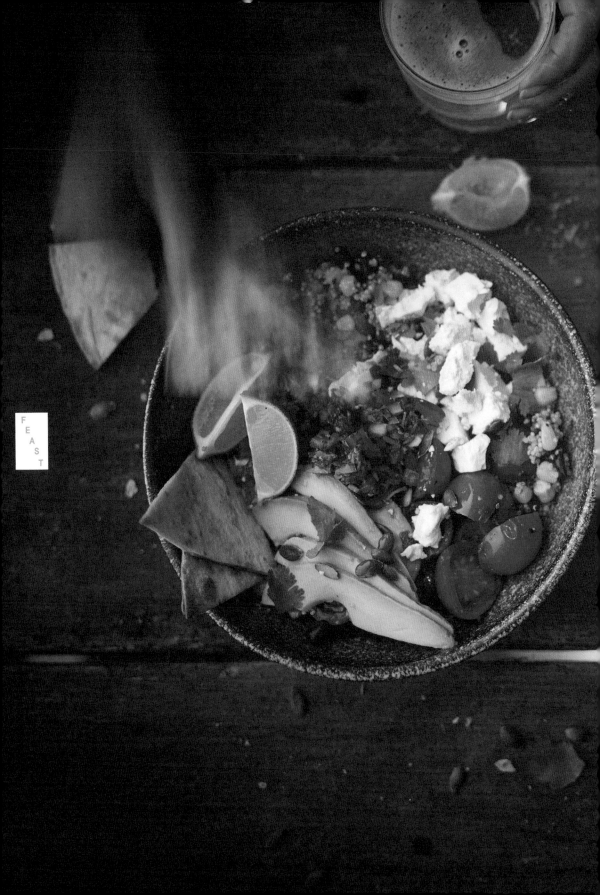

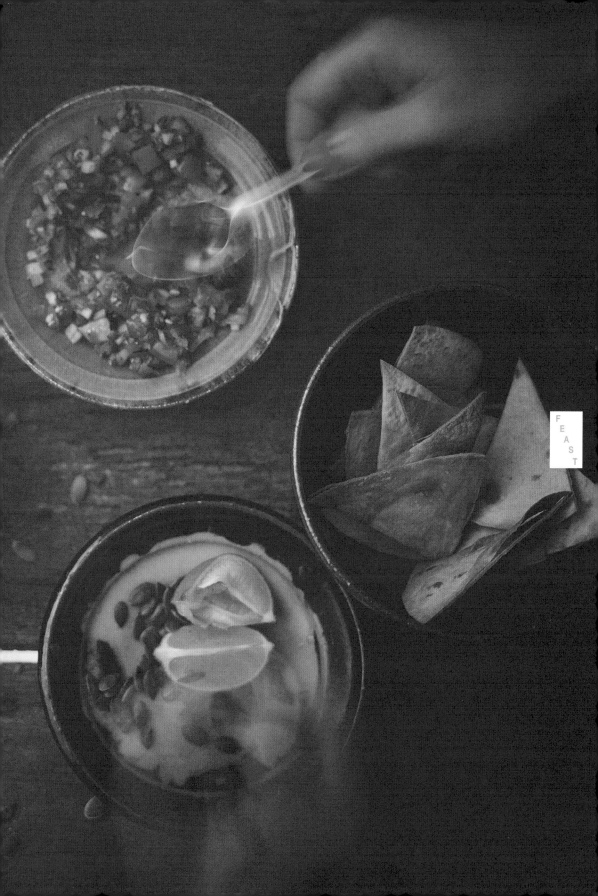

FEAST

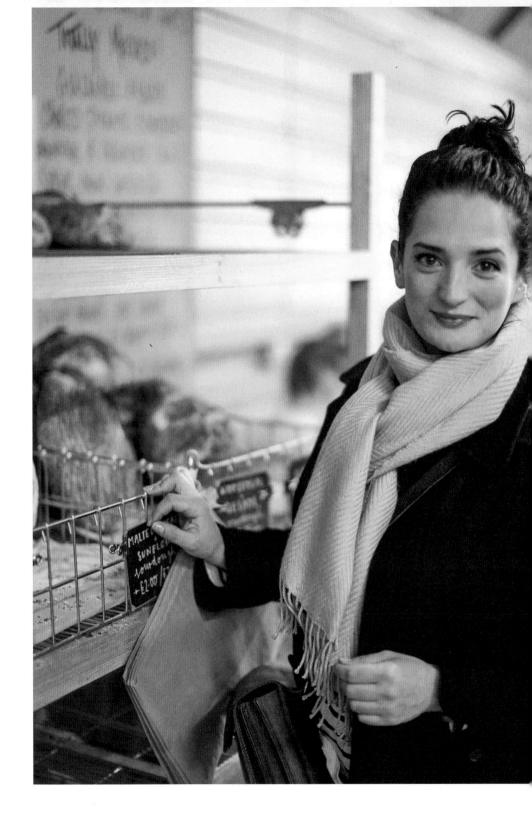

Avocado Caesar

This dressing is unbelievably delicious: it's silky, creamy, rich and punchy. You really need a ripe avocado – even verging on over-ripe – for this.

The recipe also works very well with torn-up roast chicken stirred through. If you want to add it, do so when you toss the dressing with the lettuce ribbons and give it all a really good coating.

Serves 4–6 as a starter or 2–4 as a main

---

2 baby cos or Romaine lettuce heads

1 ripe avocado

a large handful of cubes of stale sourdough bread, roasted with olive oil until golden

100g Parmesan, finely grated

For the dressing

2 anchovy fillets

2 garlic cloves

1 tsp Worcestershire sauce

1 tsp Dijon mustard

1 medium-sized ripe avocado, destoned

juice of ¼ lemon

4 tbsp olive oil

120ml good-quality shop-bought mayonnaise

large pinch of flaked sea salt

First, make the dressing. Blitz the anchovies, garlic, Worcestershire sauce and mustard in a food processor or blender. Add the avocado and lemon juice. Blitz. Add the olive oil, mayonnaise and salt. Blitz again until silky. Pour into a bowl, cover with a sheet of cling film pressed onto the surface and refrigerate until needed.

When you are just about ready to serve, remove the larger outer leaves from the lettuce and cut them into 2.5cm thick ribbons. Give the dressing a stir and if it is too thick, add a splash of water to thin it down. Put some of the dressing into a large bowl and add the lettuce ribbons. Toss well to coat.

Cut the lettuce hearts into wedges and arrange around the edges of a large serving bowl, platter or individual small plates. Pile the dressed lettuce in the centre. Slice the avocado in half and remove the stone. Scoop out the flesh and cut into bite-sized cubes, then layer on top of the dressed lettuce. Scatter over the croûtons and grated Parmesan, add extra dollops of dressing around the bowl and serve.

Seared scallops in brown butter with double Jerusalem artichoke

These scallops make an impressive and classy starter for a dinner party. Serve two in each shell, giving each guest one shell each, and put bread on the table to share. It is also exactly the sort of thing I'd like to make for a romantic dinner for two (or be made). Make the purée and crisps in advance, take a break from snogging to quickly sear the scallops, then serve with bread and champagne. Follow with a ready-to-eat pudding (like the Chocolate and PX Pots on page 253). Swit swoo.

Get scallop shells from your fishmonger, if possible, but don't feel like a failure if you have to serve them straight off a plate – it's actually easier to eat this way.

I know the recipe looks long, but you can break it down and do it in stages and it's TOTALLY worth it.

Serves 2–3

----

6 fresh scallops with roe,
    plus 2–3 shells

olive oil

1 tbsp Brown Butter
    (see page 234)

a few thyme leaves,
    for garnishing

flaked sea salt and freshly
    ground black pepper

For the crisps

100g Jerusalem artichoke

1 tbsp olive oil

flaked sea salt and freshly
    ground black pepper

For the purée

200g Jerusalem artichokes
    or parsnips

50g unsalted butter

1 tbsp double cream

½ lemon (optional)

To make the crisps, preheat the oven to 180°C/350°F/Gas mark 4 and line two baking sheets with baking parchment. Rinse the artichokes and use a mandoline to slice them really thin – 1mm at most. Drizzle with the olive oil and mix, using your fingers to make sure each slice is glistening with a light coating of the oil then lay out, in a single layer, on the prepared baking sheets. Season with black pepper and bake for 15–20 minutes, until crisp and golden. Watch them carefully, as they'll burn easily. You might need to whip some of the crisps out earlier if your oven has hot patches. When they're done, sprinkle instantly with sea salt and cool completely on a wire rack. When cooled, transfer to an airtight container and keep at room temperature for up to 12 hours.

To make the purée, peel the artichokes and cut into bite-sized pieces. Bring a pan of salted water to the boil and add the artichoke. Cook until tender. Drain, then put back in the pan and add the butter. Cover with the lid for 2 minutes to melt the butter in the residual heat. Once the butter has melted, transfer the artichoke to a food processor. Add the cream and season with a pinch of salt and pepper, then blend until totally smooth. Adjust the seasoning to taste, and add a little lemon juice if it's richer than you'd like. You can serve this straight away, or transfer to a container, leave to cool, cover and refrigerate, then reheat gently, stirring well until piping hot once you're ready to eat.

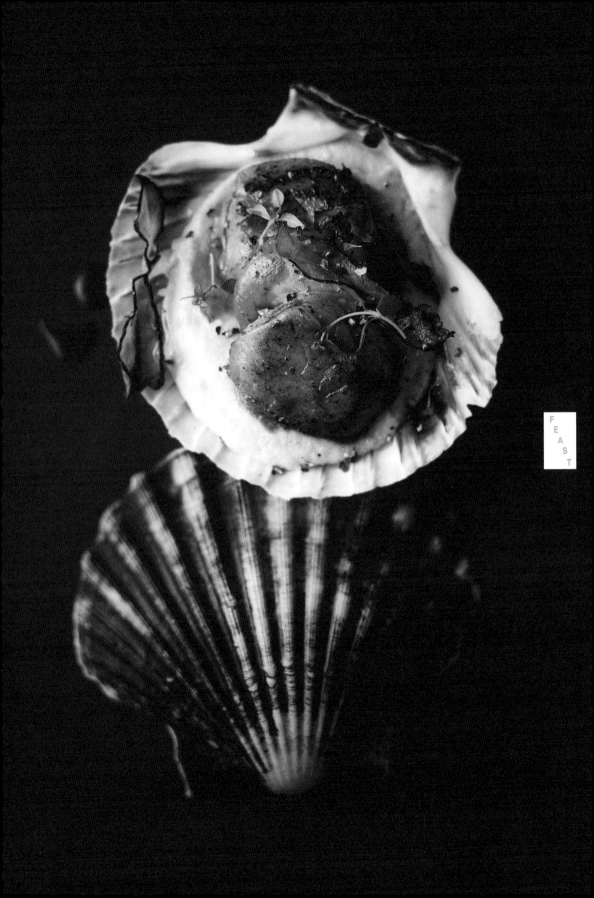

For the scallops, you'll need to work quickly and confidently – they're precious little things and need to be treated with respect. Get everything ready before you start.

Lay the scallops out on kitchen paper and dab them until totally dry. Arrange on a plate and drizzle with olive oil on both sides. Season both sides with sea salt and black pepper.

At this point, heat your purée in a pan over a low heat, stirring regularly with a rubber spatula, and get your crisps out and ready. Now you're ready to start the scallops and you're less than 4 minutes away from eating them…

Heat a large frying pan over a medium-high heat. When it's hot, place the first scallop at the top of your pan (12 o'clock). Hold down for a couple of seconds to encourage as much surface area to brown as possible. Do not shake the pan or move them once they're in; you want them to form a golden crust. Work your way around the pan, clockwise, until all the scallops are in. When you get back to the first one (at 12 o'clock), lift it gently and check that it has a nice golden crust. Gently flip it over and work your way clockwise until they're all turned over. They only need 1–2 minutes cooking in total (30 seconds to 1 minute on each side).

When they're nearly done, add the brown butter to the pan, let it foam up, then take the pan off the heat.

Remove the scallops from the pan, again, starting at 12 o'clock and working clockwise. Transfer to a plate to rest. Gently brush a little of the brown butter from the pan over the surface of each scallop.

Divide the purée between the scallop shells, if using, or plates.

Sit the scallops on top, add a few of the crisps and sprinkle with the thyme leaves. Season.

Serve with urgency.

Root vegetables, brown shrimp and soft herbs

My mate Sam Sohn-Rethel, who is head chef at my favourite restaurant, Bell's Diner in Bristol, came up with this idea. A hot restaurant kitchen in August is not the most conducive place to be developing ideas for winter dishes, but once Sam and I got chatting I was transported to those cold days when the greengrocers start filling up with all sorts of knobbly root vegetables. We discussed a few ideas, then Sam's eyes lit up as he hit upon this combo.

Salsify is in season from around October to January, so you have plenty of time to hunt some down. But, if you can"t get hold of any, you can use Jerusalem artichokes, celeriac, Anya potatoes or regular new potatoes will do. Heritage carrots or beetroot may work, too. You get the idea. Mix it up or just use one type. If you're using red beetroot, just cook them separately in a second pan or you'll turn everything red.

Serves 4, as a starter

—

800g root veg (see above)

juice of 1 lemon

100g salted butter

fresh nutmeg

a few thyme sprigs

100g brown shrimp, cooked and peeled

handful of tarragon, leaves picked

handful of dill, leaves picked

lemon wedges, for squeezing

sea salt and freshly grated black pepper

Start by peeling your veg. Fill a bowl with cold water and squeeze in some fresh lemon juice.

Cut the veg into bite-sized pieces, at various angles to create maximum surface areas. As you cut, place the pieces in the lemon water. (This stops the root veg from going brown while you prep the rest.)

Bring a pan of salted water to the boil over high heat, and add the vegetables. Reduce the heat to medium-high and simmer for 5 minutes. Drain well.

Melt the butter in a large pan over a medium-high heat until foaming. Add the vegetables and season well with salt, pepper and a good grating of nutmeg. Add in the sprigs of thyme and spoon the butter all over the veg. Turn the heat right down to low. Keep the veg in one layer and keep basting regularly with the butter, until tender. Depending on the veg used, this will take between 20 and 45 minutes. Using tongs, turn the veg over a couple of times during the cooking. Taste for seasoning.

Remove from the heat and divide between four plates. Sprinkle over the brown shrimp, plenty of tarragon and dill and a good squeeze of lemon. Drizzle over the browned butter from the pan and serve.

FEAST

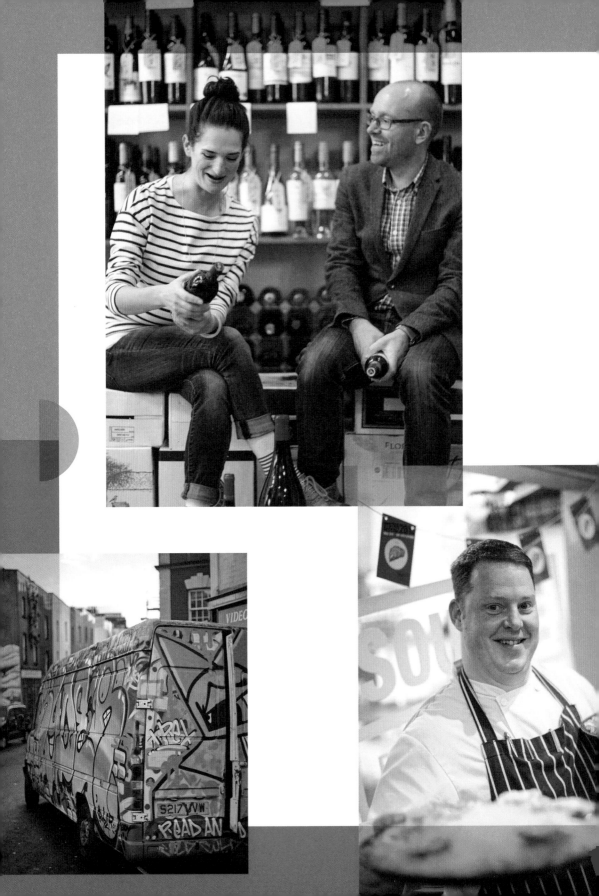

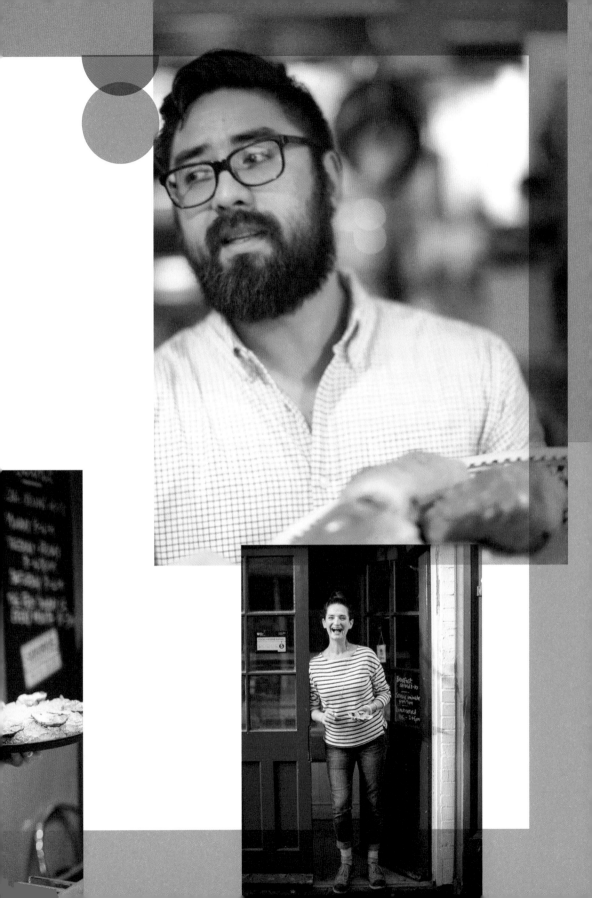

Blue cheese polenta with mushrooms and hazelnuts

You know those days after Christmas when there are various leftover bits of cheese and the end of a bag of mixed nuts? This is the perfect way to use everything up.

You can use all sorts of cheese in this if you don't want to use a blue. A strong cheddar would work well, as would simply using extra Parmesan.

Serves 2
—

240ml full-fat milk

1 bay leaf

1 garlic clove, smashed

1 rosemary sprig

5 black peppercorns

10g whole hazelnuts

1 tbsp olive oil

1 banana shallot, cut into 5mm slices

2 large field or Portobello mushrooms, cut into 5mm slices

small bunch thyme sprigs

2 tbsp fino sherry or dry white wine

10g butter

75g quick-cook polenta

40g blue cheese

10g Parmesan, finely grated

flaked sea salt and freshly ground black pepper

A few thyme leaves, to garnish

To make the wet polenta, combine the milk, bay leaf, garlic, thyme and rosemary sprigs and black peppercorns with 240ml water in a pan. Set over a high heat and bring to the boil. Turn off the heat and leave to infuse for 30 minutes.

Meanwhile, toast the hazelnuts in a dry frying pan over a medium heat then roughly chop.

Wipe out the pan and heat 1 tablespoon of olive oil. Add the shallot, season and gently fry over a low heat, stirring frequently. Once they are golden brown, add the mushrooms, thyme and the sherry or wine. Turn heat up until the booze has bubbled away then add the butter. Cook over a gentle heat, stirring frequently.

Strain the milk and herb mixture for the polenta back into a clean saucepan and discard the solids. Set over a medium heat and bring to the boil. While continuously whisking, pour in the polenta in a slow and steady stream. Be careful, it's very likely to spit. After a minute or so crumble in the blue cheese and the Parmesan and beat until all the cheese has melted.

Take off the heat and season to taste. Add more milk if it's too thick (it should be the consistency of potato purée).

Divide the polenta between two plates and top with the mushrooms and thyme leaves.

Serve immediately.

This is also great with extra blue cheese on the top, or even a poached egg.

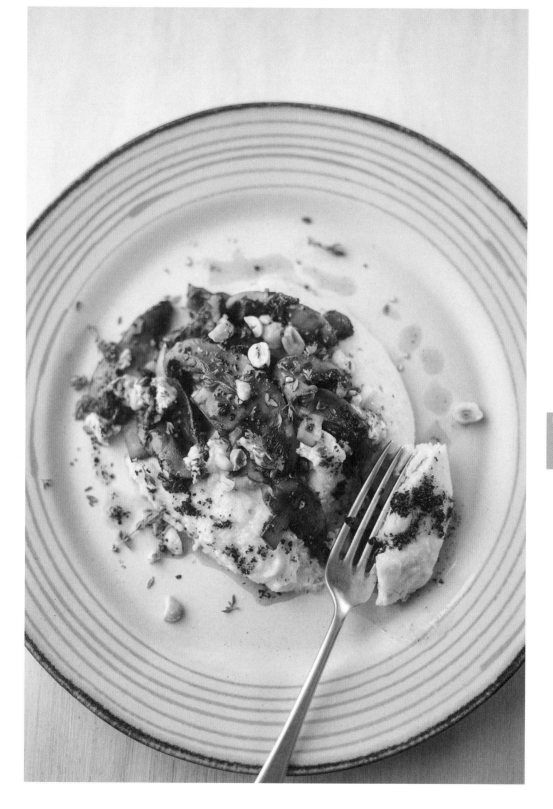

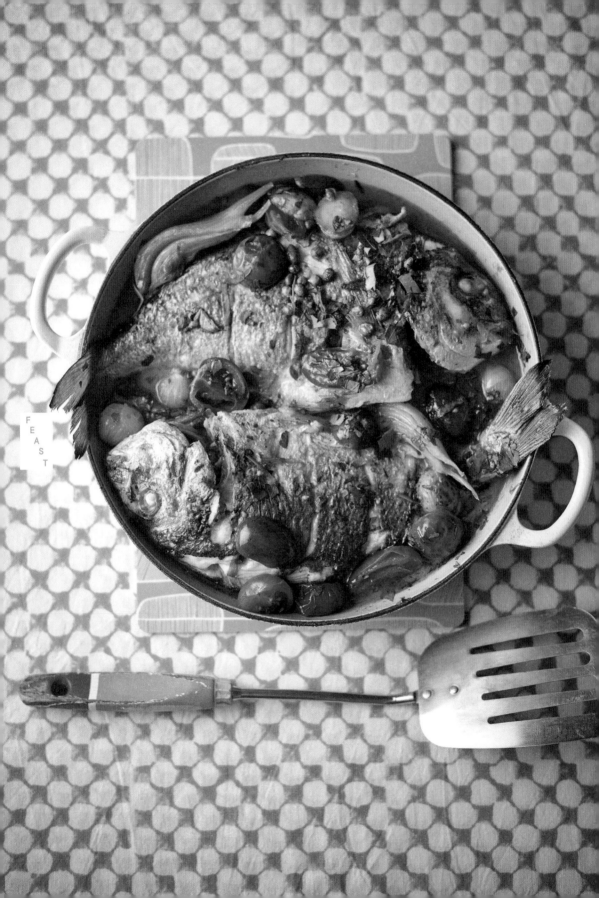

FEAST

Sea bream in crazy water with fennel and potatoes

This is a classic dish, which is translated from 'Orata all'acqua pazza'. The 'crazy water' is the hot spicy tomato sauce that you slip your fish in to cook. There are loads of recipes out there, but this is my version, a one-pot dinner for two.

Serves 2

---

1 fennel bulb

4 tbsp olive oil

1 tsp unsalted butter

6 cooked new potatoes, thickly sliced

2 x whole sea bream, cleaned (ask your fishmonger)

2 garlic cloves, finely sliced

1 bird's eye chilli, finely sliced

400g mixed tomatoes, cut in half if large

4 tbsp white wine

1 heaped tbsp capers, drained and rinsed well

flat-leaf parsley, finely chopped, plus extra roughly chopped for the garnish

extra-virgin olive oil, for drizzling

flaked sea salt and freshly ground black pepper

Cut the fronds from the fennel and set aside. Slice the bulb into six wedges, keeping the root intact.

Heat 2 tablespoons of olive oil and the butter in a large frying pan (that will hold both fish comfortably) over a medium heat. When the butter starts to brown, add the fennel wedges and cooked potato. Cook for 4–5 minutes on one side until nicely browned before turning and browning the other side, until they start to collapse. Try not to move the veg around too much – you want them to caramelise.

Carefully, using tongs, remove the veg to a plate and set aside.

Add the remaining olive oil to the pan and heat over a medium heat.

Slash each fish three times on each side, at an angle, cutting just a couple of millimetres deep.

Slip the fish into the hot oil and cook for 5 minutes, until they start to brown. Flip over and add the garlic to the pan. Cook for a further 1 minute, then add the chilli and tomatoes. Return the fennel and potato to the pan, tucking it into the gaps around the fish.

Pour over the wine and let it bubble for 1 minute, then pour in 100ml water. Bring to the boil over a medium-high heat. Season well with salt and pepper, and put on the lid. Simmer for 15 minutes, until the fish is cooked through.

Transfer the fish to a plate and set aside.

Add the capers and parsley to the pan and boil vigorously for 1 minute. Turn off the heat.

Slip the fish back into the pan and drizzle with olive oil. Garnish with the roughly chopped parsley and take the whole pan to the table.

Bloody Mary prawn salad

Jamie Oliver deserves the credit for this idea. He serves a big platter of little gem 'cups' filled with prawns, shrimps and smoked salmon. It's an impressive party platter, and you can make enough for a big group as easily as doing it for just two.

Serves 2

—

For the dressing

80g tomato passata

¼ tbsp mayonnaise

¼ tsp Worcestershire sauce

½ tsp tabasco, to taste

¼ tsp creamed horseradish

¼ tsp vodka

sea salt and freshly ground black pepper

For the salad

50g little gem lettuce

50g radicchio

20g fennel, finely sliced

140g cooked king prawns

a few sprigs of dill

6g cress or micro herbs

5g celery leaves

lemon wedges

F
A
S
T

Blitz all the dressing ingredients in a bowl, or whisk together well.

Separate the leaves of the little gem and lay them on a serving plate. Layer around the radicchio and fennel. Top with the prawns and garnish with the dill, cress and celery leaves.

Splatter some of the dressing over the salad and serve the rest on the side.

Season then serve, squeezing the lemon juice over the whole salad before eating.

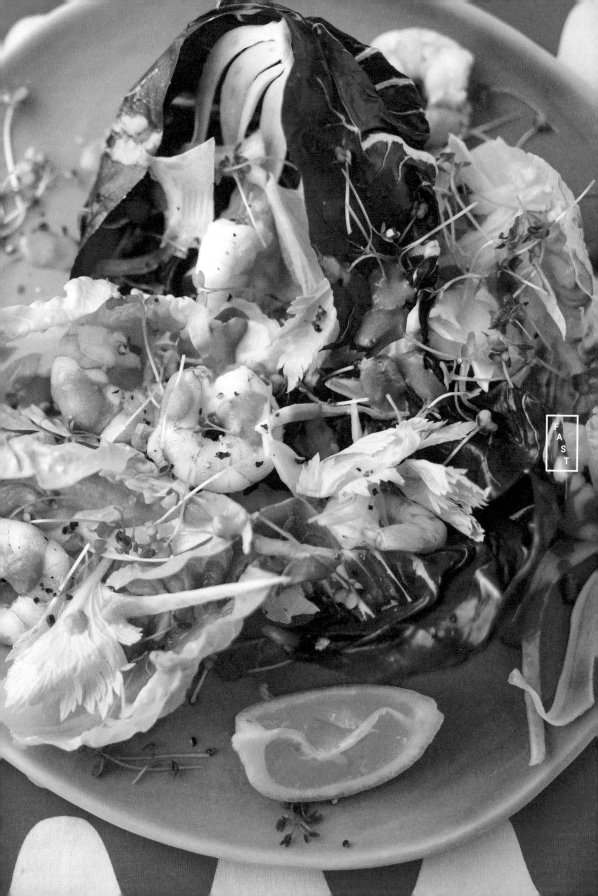

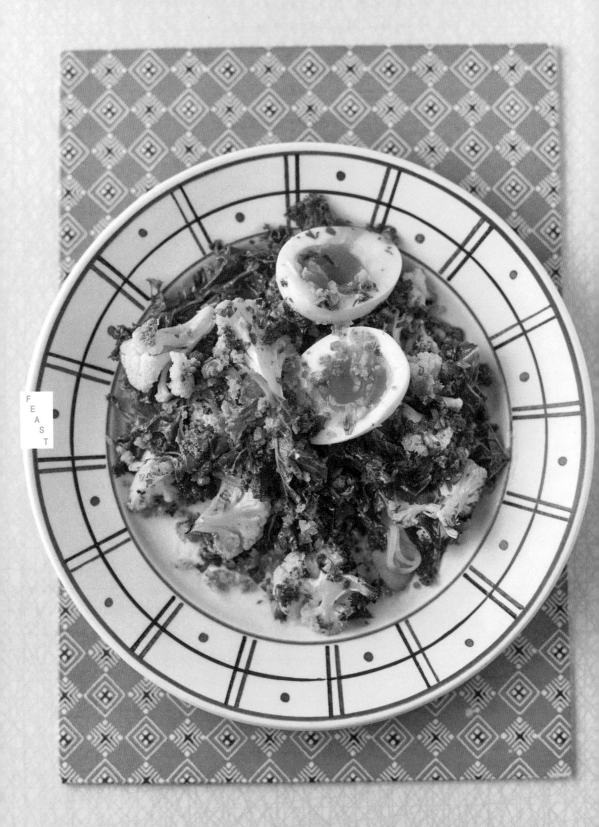

Roasted cauliflower meunière

Meunière (meaning miller's wife) sauce is a variation on a brown butter sauce. There are different versions of this, but parsley and lemon are fixed. It is usually served with fish dredged in seasoned flour (hence the miller bit), but the sauce goes really well with roasted cauliflower, too.

An indulgent way to serve the humble cauliflower, it makes a really special dinner for two. It's a little tricky to scale up, so keep this one for when there's just you and someone else who deserves a treat. If you can't eat gluten, swap the breadcrumbs for roughly chopped hazelnuts to give you the vital element of crunch.

Serves 2

1 small cauliflower, broken into florets

2 tbsp olive oil, plus extra for drizzling

2 tbsp sourdough breadcrumbs

2 tsp Wyfe of Bath cheese or Parmesan, finely grated

2 eggs

2 garlic cloves, thinly sliced

2 handfuls of kale, prepared according to page 17

1 lemon, zest finely grated and quartered and deseeded

4 tbsp Brown Butter (see page 234)

1 banana shallot, thinly sliced

1 heaped tbsp roughly chopped capers

2 tbsp chopped flat-leaf parsley

2 tbsp Bath Blue cheese or other creamy blue cheese such as Cashel Blue, crumbled (optional)

sea salt and freshly ground black pepper

Preheat the oven to 220°C/425°F/Gas mark 7.

Arrange the cauliflower on a roasting tray lined with baking parchment. Drizzle with 1 tablespoon of olive oil, season with salt and roast for about 20 minutes, until cooked and golden.

Heat the remaining olive oil in a frying pan. Add the breadcrumbs and season. Shake regularly and fry the crumbs over a medium heat, for a couple of minutes, until evenly toasted. Remove from the heat and tip into a bowl. Add the Wyfe of Bath or Parmesan cheese and stir well. Wipe out the pan.

Boil the eggs according to the 6-minute egg method (see page 16), but leave the eggs to cook for an extra 20 seconds.

Meanwhile, back to the pan. Add a drizzle of oil and fry the garlic and kale over a medium heat for a couple of minutes. Add a little water and stir in the lemon zest. Remove from the heat and transfer to a bowl. Cover and set aside in a warm place. Wipe out the pan.

Next, make the sauce. Melt a knob of brown butter in the pan. Remove from the heat and stir in the shallot, capers, parsley, lemon juice and season to taste.

Place some cauliflower on the plates. Add the kale, cheesy crumbs, egg and finish with the sauce. Crumble Bath Blue (if using) around the plate.

F
E
A
S
T

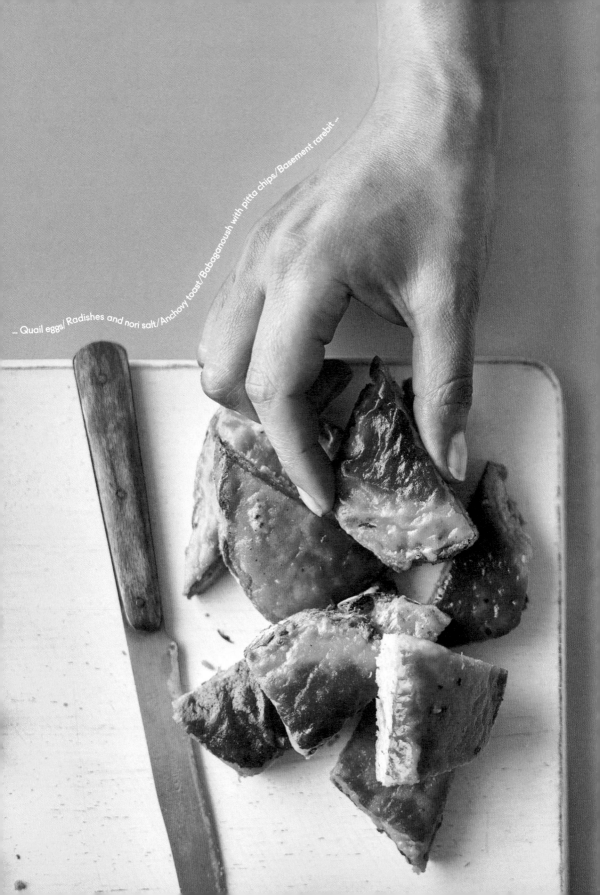

... Quail eggs/ Radishes and nori salt/ Anchovy toast/ Babaganoush with pitta chips/ Basement rarebit ...

Nibbles

Babaganoush
with pitta chips

Pitta chips are the best way to make a big pile of homemade nibbles for a matter of pence. You can flavour them with all sorts of things – just sprinkle on before baking. Curry powder-flavoured pitta chips dipped into mango chutney mixed with yoghurt (and served with beer) was a regular favourite in my twenties. My taste buds have grown up, but that sweet, spicy combo still tastes great.

Here is a bit of a classier combo. I love anything smoky and babaganoush gets its delicious charred flavour from the first step of blackening the aubergine. Do not rush this bit. You want the aubergine to look totally RUINED. Then, it's ready.

Serves 4-6
—

1 large aubergine
1 tbsp tahini
juice of ½ lemon
1 garlic clove, crushed
1 tbsp chopped mint
1 tbsp chopped flat-leaf
  parsley
smoked salt
1 tbsp argan oil, or your best
  extra-virgin olive oil

For the pitta chips
6 pitta breads
olive oil, for drizzling
3 tsp za'atar (see page 228)

First, make the babaganoush by blistering the aubergine directly over a gas flame, on a barbecue, gas hob, or in a foil-lined tray under a preheated hot grill. Keep turning until the aubergine is totally blackened, blistered and really collapsing, about 30 minutes.

Remove and allow to cool.

When cool, split the aubergine in half, scoop out the flesh, put in a sieve over a bowl and set aside for 30 minutes. Discard the blackened skin.

Preheat the oven to 180°C/350°F/Gas mark 4.

Mash the aubergine gently. I do this with a spoon, using the edge of it to break up the longer strands of aubergine flesh to make a purée.

In a bowl, mix the tahini with the lemon juice. Add the crushed garlic and most of the herbs, setting some aside to garnish. Season well with smoked salt.

Add the aubergine to the mix and give it a good stir. Taste. Adjust the lemon juice, tahini and seasoning where necessary.

Next, make the pitta chips. Toast your pittas for 30 seconds, until they puff up. Use a big pair of kitchen scissors to cut the pitta breads widthways into 8–10 strips, being careful of the steam.

Split the two halves apart and lay the strips, rough side up, on a baking sheet, making sure they don't overlap. Drizzle them all with a little olive oil and sprinkle evenly with za'atar.

Bake in the preheated oven for about 5 minutes, or until golden brown. Remove and set aside to cool; the chips will crisp up as they cool down.

Just before serving, top the babaganoush with the remaining herbs and pour over a slick of oil. Arrange the babaganoush in a bowl on a platter and have pitta chips on the side for dipping.

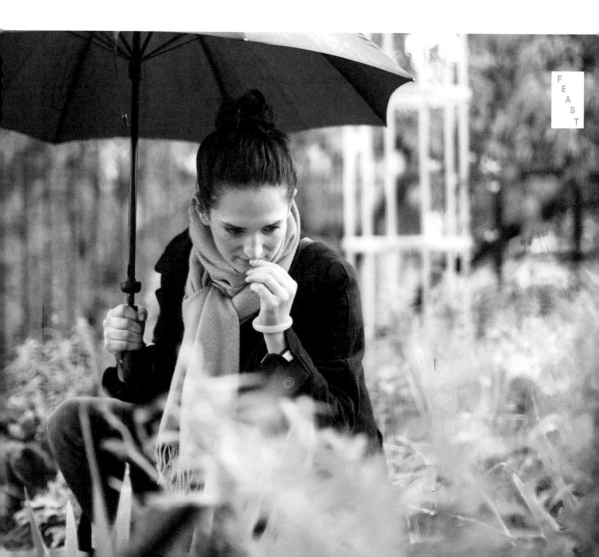

Pan con tomate

I love Spain. I've been loads and spend my time there generally eating, drinking and smiling.

Bread, oil, tomato, salt. The simple things are so often the best and this dish not only makes a great breakfast, it also works really well as a pre-dinner snack. Simply cut up into bite-sized pieces and serve along with slices of Manchego cheese, a cold glass of fino sherry or a glass of Cava. You'll be feeling those holiday vibes before you know it.

This is my good friend José Pizarro's technique. He owns some of London's very best Spanish restaurants and is the most Spanish man I know, so I reckon you won't get much better than this recipe.

Serves 2

---

4 slices of bread (José recommends a Spanish bread called Pan de Cristal, which is very similar to ciabatta)

2 garlic cloves, peeled

best-quality extra-virgin olive oil, for drizzling

2 very ripe tomatoes, coarsely grated

flaked sea salt and freshly ground black pepper

Preheat the oven to 180°C/350°F/Gas mark 4.

Place the bread on a baking tray and toast in the oven for about 3–4 minutes, or until golden brown.

Rub the garlic cloves directly against the rough surface of both sides of the toasted bread.

Pile the grated tomatoes onto your bread and liberally drizzle with olive oil.

Sprinkle with sea salt flakes and pepper. Serve.

Spicy roasted chickpeas

These crisp, spicy chickpeas are fantastic to nibble on with drinks, especially beer. They're baked rather than deep-fried and they contain loads of protein. Eat them on their own or mix with nuts, or sprinkle over salads or roast vegetables.

Serves 2

1 x 400g tin chickpeas, drained and rinsed

2 tsp olive oil

¼ tsp each of the following:

    ground cumin

    ground coriander

    ground cinnamon

    Turkish chilli flakes

    sweet smoked paprika

    flaked sea salt

Preheat the oven to 200°C/400°F/Gas mark 6.

Spread the chickpeas out on a dry, clean tea towel. Pat really dry and tumble onto a large baking tray lined with baking parchment. Bake for about 45 minutes, giving the chickpeas a good shake after 20 minutes, or until they're crunchy throughout.

Combine the spices in a small bowl.

Remove the roasted chickpeas from the oven and immediately, while still hot, toss in the oil and the spice mix.

F
E
A
S
T

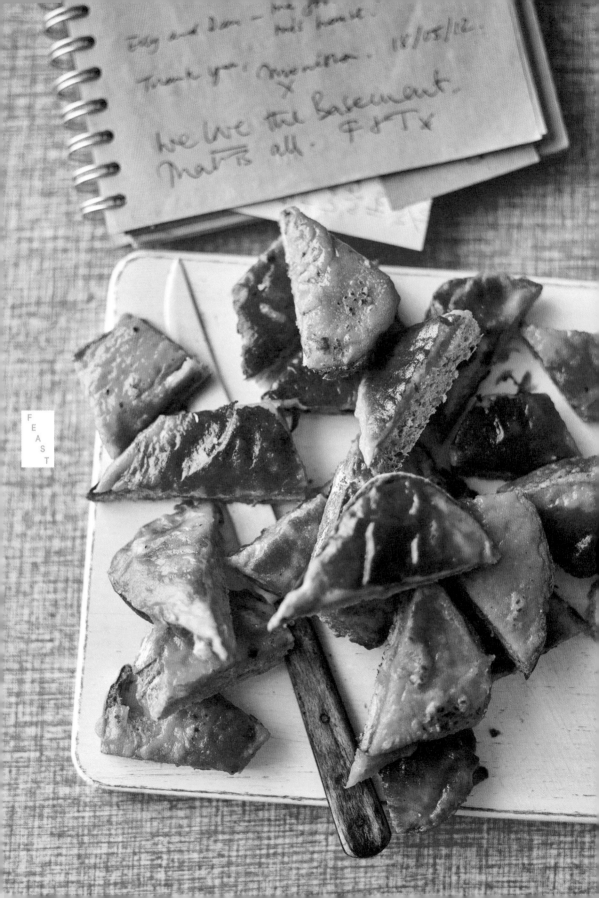

Basement rarebit

This was always the final course at The Basement, the supper club I ran with Dan in Bristol. We used to serve seven courses and finishing on a savoury mouthful was always a popular touch. What started as the classic Mark Hix recipe from *The Ivy Cookbook* got a West Country twist and became a great way to showcase local producers and friends. Make the cheesy mixture up to two days in advance, then all you need to do is spread it on toast and grill it when you're ready to serve. Hand them out with glasses of port and revel in the Edwardian dinner-party vibes.

Serves 4-6

150g good-quality strong Cheddar, grated

3 medium egg yolks (keep the whites to make the Italian Meringues on page 248)

1 tbsp Worcestershire sauce

1 tsp English mustard

6 drops of Tabasco

2 tbsp stout (we used Bristol Beer Factory Milk Stout)

8 slices of sourdough bread, cut 1cm thick

flaked sea salt and freshly ground black pepper

In a bowl, combine the cheese with the eggs, Worcestershire sauce, mustard, Tabasco and stout and season with salt and pepper to make a thick paste.

You can now store this paste in the fridge until you're ready to serve.

To serve, preheat your grill. Toast your bread on both sides.

Spread the mixture evenly all over the slices, right up to the edges. If any bread is showing, it'll burn. Put onto a grill tray lined with foil. Grill for 4–5 minutes, or until the cheese is golden and blistered in blackened patches.

Move the slices onto a board and cut into bite-sized pieces.

Serve immediately.

FEAST

Cider-battered onions

Before we started The Basement and before we even met, Dan was writing a food blog, 'EssexEating'. His way with words is unique and funny. He wrote up one of our most popular dishes back in 2012 and I am going to leave it to him to explain:

'This is a quick recipe we served a number of times at The Basement supper club as a nibble and it's superb, ridiculously easy to knock out, cheap and absolutely delicious. The flavour combination of deep-fried, hot-battered onions and the sharp tang of the onion salt is cracking.

Just a couple of onions is enough to feed a whole horde, it's amazing, so it's tres frugal too and therefore suitable recession eating.'

Serves 10
—
2 large Spanish onions

vegetable oil, for deep-frying

plain flour, for dusting

flaked sea salt and freshly
    ground black pepper

For the onion salt
2 tbsp sea salt
2 tbsp dried onions
    (available
    from supermarkets)

For the cider batter
80g self-raising flour
120ml dry cider

First, make the onion salt by blitzing the ingredients together in a food processor until you have a fine, salty dust.

Slice the onions in half and cut into 1cm thick slices. Separate the slices.

Next, make the batter by whisking the flour and cider in a bowl until thick and smooth. Season and leave to rest for 30 minutes.

Heat the vegetable oil to 180°C/350°F in a deep-fat fryer, or large pan.

Season the flour for dusting, then toss the onions in the flour. Dip the coated pieces of onion into the batter and, in batches, drop the onions into the hot oil. Deep-fry until golden and crisp.

Remove and drain on kitchen paper before sprinkling straight away with the onion salt.

Little roasted spuds with roasted red pepper sauce

These are a simple and cheap canapé. I love dunking these into the Roasted Red Pepper Sauce on page 229 but a garlicky mayo would be stunning, too. You need to serve them straight away, so get the sauce made up to two days before, parboil the potatoes up to 24 hours in advance, then just stick them in the oven half an hour before you want to serve them. Join the party, then pop back to the kitchen to grate the Parmesan over the top and re-emerge with a pile of hot, cheesy potatoes. You'll be mega popular.

Serves 6

1kg new potatoes (cut any that are bigger than a ping-pong ball in half)

1 tbsp olive oil

1 tbsp balsamic vinegar

1 tbsp sesame seeds

20g Parmesan

1 quantity Roasted Red Pepper Sauce (see page 229)

flaked sea salt and freshly ground black pepper

Preheat the oven to 220°C/430°F/Gas mark 7.

Put the potatoes in a large pan and fill with water. Bring to the boil and cook the potatoes for 10 minutes, over a medium heat, until just tender, but firm when pierced with a tip of a knife.

Drain and tip into a roasting tray. Drizzle with the oil and vinegar and toss well. Sprinkle with the sesame seeds and season well.

Roast the potatoes for 25–30 minutes, until they're nicely golden.

Stick a cocktail stick into each potato, pile up in a bowl and finely grate the Parmesan over them. Serve with a bowl of the Roasted Red Pepper Sauce for dipping.

FEAST

Pink popcorn

You can make popcorn at home in less than five minutes and you don't need a microwave. You can also control your portion size if you avoid pre-packaged microwave popcorn, you save on packaging and it's loads cheaper, too.

Beetroot powder and coconut oil was a surprise hit combination when I started playing around with new flavour ideas. It's a little sweet, but not overly so, and there's no added sugar or salt. The coconut oil gives the popcorn a coconutty taste, and there is the added bonus of it being a crazy bright pink. Barbara Cartland would love this stuff.

One caveat is that it will stain your fingers. That's kind of the deal with beetroot, though. By the way, it won't taste of beetroot.

Makes a huge bowlful, like an XL tub from the cinema

—

2 tbsp coconut oil
100g popcorn kernels

3 tsp beetroot powder (available from Indian supermarkets or online)

Heat the coconut oil in a large lidded pan, over a medium heat, until it is totally liquid.

Pour the kernels into the hot oil and put the lid on. Turn the heat right down as low as it will go.

Stay nearby and listen carefully. Shake the pan well (holding the lid on) every 30 seconds or so.

After a couple of minutes, the kernels will start to pop. As soon as this happens, stop and remove the pan from the heat.

Sprinkle half the beetroot powder evenly over the popcorn, shake well, then add the rest.

Pour into a large serving bowl and eat.

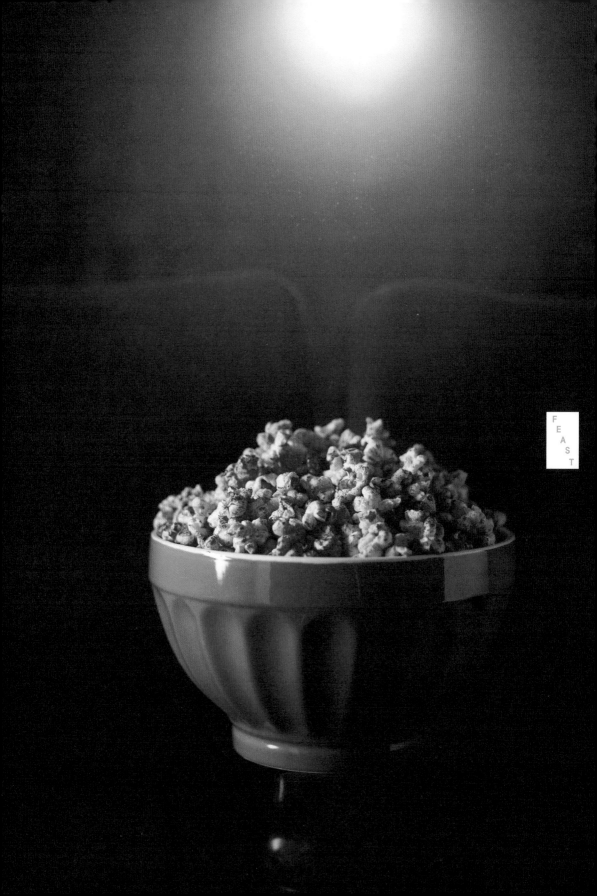

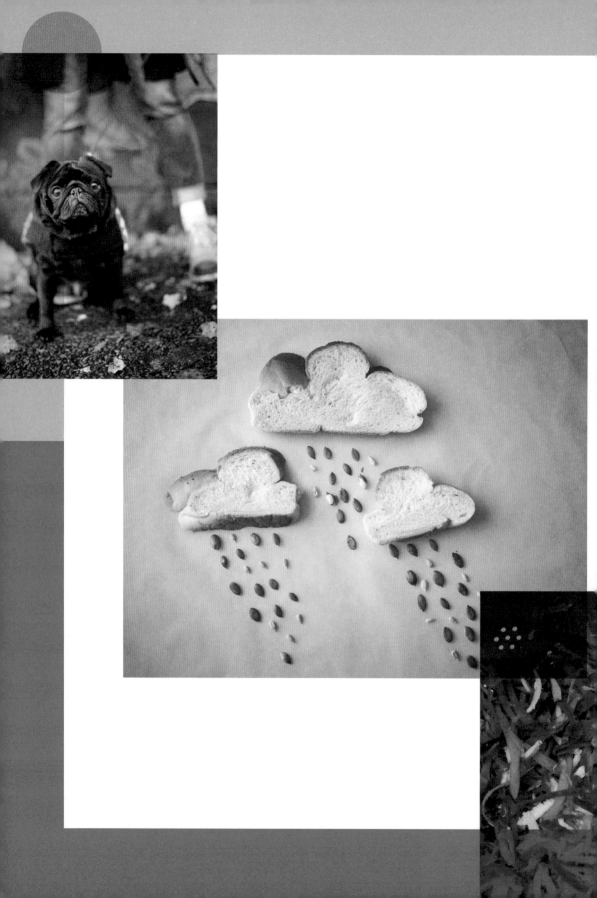

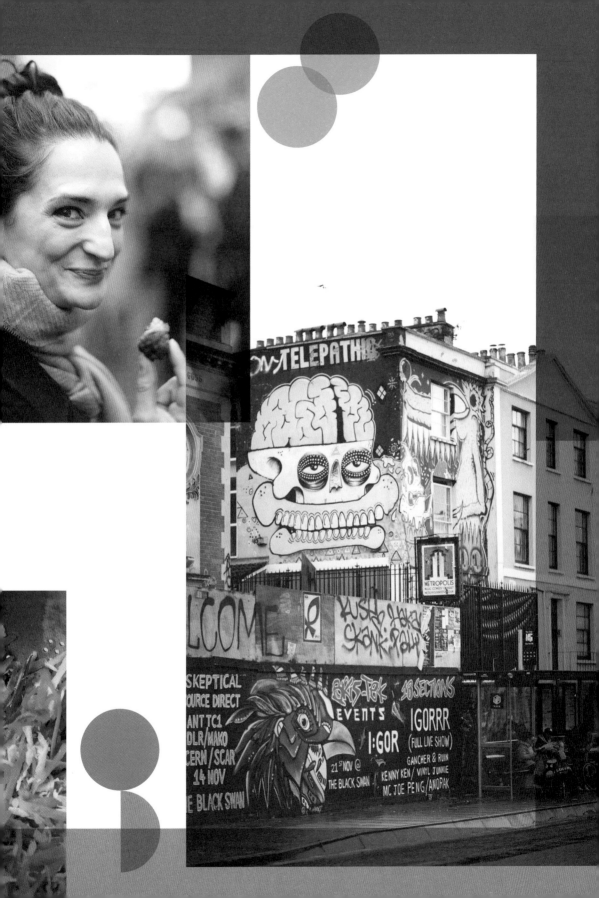

Smoked mackerel and horseradish pâté

Obviously you can use this in sandwiches (best with little gem, toasted seeds and gherkins on poppy seed bloomer), but I make it most often for parties. Serve spread on a mini oatcake garnished with a few picked thyme or dill leaves for a fabulous canapé. Or put the whole bowl out with a couple of knives stuck in, chunks of fresh bread, some watercress and a bowl of cornichons and let guests help themselves.

Makes 20 mini canapes or 1 big bowl-full

—

350g smoked
    mackerel fillets

150g cream cheese

3 tsp horseradish

75ml double cream
    (or use crème fraîche
    for more tang)

juice of ¼ lemon

flaked sea salt and freshly
    ground black pepper

F
A
S
T

Peel the skin off the mackerel fillets, then flake the fish into a bowl. Look out for any small bones and pick them out if you spot one.

Add the cream cheese, horseradish, cream and lemon juice and mix well. You want it well combined, but with a few chunks of mackerel.

Season to taste and refrigerate for 1 hour before serving.

Anchovy toast

An umami bomb to eat with fino, beer or fizz, these are always really popular as pre-dinner snacks. They're ready in minutes and use mostly storecupboard ingredients. Use marinated white anchovy fillets if you want a mild taste, or the ones packed in oil or salt if you want a stronger hit. Swap the anchovies for black olives, roughly chopped, if you're veggie or vegan.

Serves 6–8

—

6 slices of sourdough bread

olive oil, for drizzling

2 garlic cloves, peeled and halved lengthways

flaked sea salt

2 grilled red peppers from a jar, cut into thin strips

12 anchovy fillets, halved lengthways

2 tbsp mini capers

a few sprigs of flat-leaf parsley

1 tbsp toasted fennel seeds

zest of 1 lemon, finely grated

Chargrill or toast your bread slices. While still hot, drizzle with olive oil and rub a garlic clove all over both sides of each toast. Sprinkle with salt. Cut the toast into bite-sized pieces and put on a serving plate.

Pile a few strips of red pepper on top of each slice of toast and tangle an anchovy fillet in amongst the pepper. Add a couple of capers, a parsley leaf and a sprinkle of fennel seeds onto each toast. Just before serving, grate over a tiny bit of lemon zest.

F
E
A
S
T

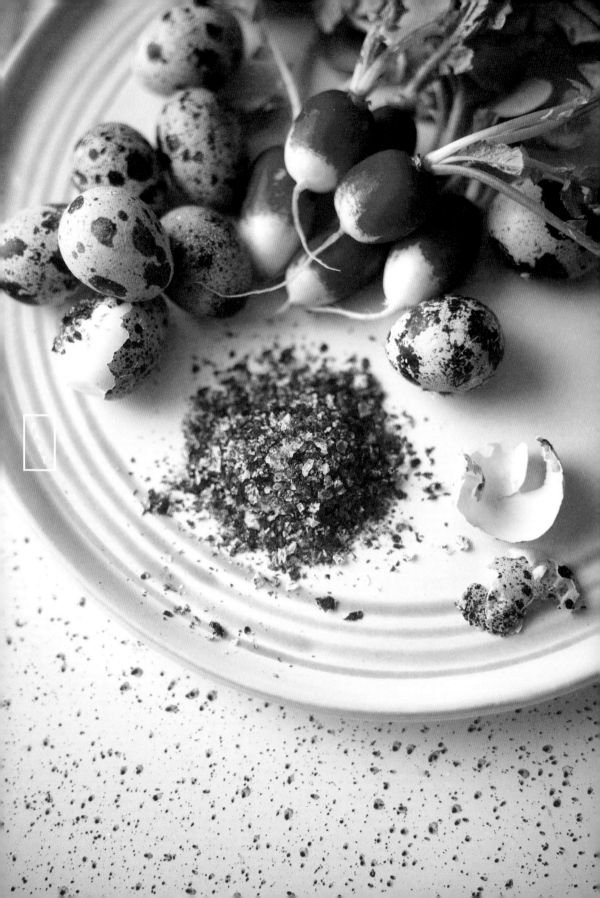

Radishes and nori salt

Radishes are ridiculously low in calories. Well, they are basically crunchy water, aren't they? You can munch your way through loads of them on a fast day which them great to have on hand for snacking on.

The nori salt also works well with 6-minute eggs (page 16) and blanched asparagus. Also try the za'atar on page 228 for dipping radishes in. If it's not a fast day, butter, salt and radishes is a heavenly snack. If the butter is soft enough to drag the radish through, do that. If it's cold and hard, cut a little slit in the radish and slip a thin slice of butter in the crevice. Dip the whole lot in salt.

Serves 1
—
10 radishes (breakfast
    or regular)
1 sheet of dried nori seaweed
flaked sea salt

Wash the radishes and slice them in half. Keep the leaves on if they have them.

Using a pair of tongs, hold the nori sheet over a gas flame until it crinkles – this will take a matter of seconds.

Put into a spice grinder and blitz until you have a fine dust. Measure an equal quantity of salt and mix with the ground nori.

Pile the nori-salt mixture in a little heap on your plate and dip the radishes into it.

F
A
S
T

Quail eggs

Quail eggs are tiny and cook really fast. They're also very low in calories and look ace. Fast-day winners, I reckon.

To boil

For quail eggs that have a creamy but set yolk, simply put in a small pan. Boil the kettle. Pour the just-boiled water into the pan, trying to avoid pouring it directly onto the eggs.

Cook over a medium-low heat for 45 seconds. Put the timer on, you need to be very accurate.

As soon as the timer is up, whip the pan off the heat and pour the hot water away while holding back the eggs with a spoon. Blast the eggs with cold water until they're totally cold.

Tap them gently all over to crack the shell. Roll the egg gently on the counter and the shell will start to break away. Peel the shell away gently with the pad of your thumb.

Dip them into	Serve with
Celery salt	Radishes
Smoked salt	Cherry tomatoes
Flaked sea salt with chipotle chilli	Crudités
Nori salt (see above)	Breadsticks

SNACK

C K options

F
A
S
T

for under 100 kcal

86

2 wholegrain rice cakes

+ 50g chopped tomato

+ 30g cottage cheese

+ a few sprigs of basil, seasoned well

88

A 6-minute egg

+ 50g steamed asparagus spears to dip into it

99

1 glass of ice-cold oat milk (150ml) blitzed with 10g raw cacao powder

+ a couple of cubes of ice

37

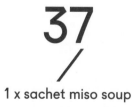

1 x sachet miso soup

+ 10g spring onion

22

60g celery sticks

+ 100g Pico de Gallo (see page 235)

99

100g little gem lettuce, cut into wedges,

+ topped with 10g very finely grated Parmesan

+ 1 teaspoon extra-virgin olive oil, lots of pepper

+ 1 teaspoon sherry vinegar

F
A
S
T

68

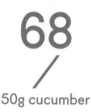

50g cucumber

+ 10g spring onion, cut into thin sticks and then wrapped in a small rice-paper wrapper

+ dipped in 10g hoisin sauce

Hummous four ways

All these recipes are made in the same way: simply chuck everything in a food processor and blitz until totally smooth. Taste and adjust as necessary, not just the seasoning but the balance of lemon juice, tahini and olive oil. Add some warm water if the hummous is too stiff. If I'm serving hummous as a dip, I make it thinner than if it's going in a sandwich. Make your hummous wet and it'll only make a soggy sandwich. Nobody wants that.

Basic hummous

1 x 400g tin chickpeas, drained and rinsed
1 garlic clove
1 tbsp tahini
1 tbsp lemon juice
1 tbsp olive oil
sea salt and freshly ground black
    pepper, to taste

Butternut squash hummous

Great on toast with feta crumbled on top and a few pumpkin seeds.

200g butternut squash, cubed
1 x 400g tin chickpeas, drained and rinsed
1 garlic clove
2 tbsp tahini
1 tbsp lemon juice
1 tsp sea salt
¼ tsp smoked paprika
freshly ground black pepper, to taste
pumpkin seeds, for garnishing

Toss the butternut squash in a dash of olive oil, season with salt and pepper and roast at 180°C/350°F/Gas mark 4 for 40 minutes, or until soft and beginning to char. Put everything in the food processor and blitz. Garnish with the pumpkin seeds.

Beetroot and dill hummous

Really good on toast, topped with brown shrimps and nutmeg.

250g cooked beetroot
1 x 400g tin chickpeas, drained and rinsed
2 tbsp olive oil
1 garlic clove
2 tbsp tahini
1 tbsp lemon juice
2 tbsp chopped dill
1 tsp sea salt, or to taste
freshly ground black pepper, to taste

To garnish
dill sprigs
Greek yoghurt

Avocado hummous

Great with the pitta chips on page 198.

1 x 400g tin chickpeas, drained and rinsed
1½ tbsp tahini
1 tbsp lime juice
1 garlic clove
pinch of ground cumin
2 ripe avocados, peeled and destoned
smoked salt and freshly ground
    black pepper, to taste

To garnish
smoked olive oil
Turkish chilli flakes
toasted cumin seeds

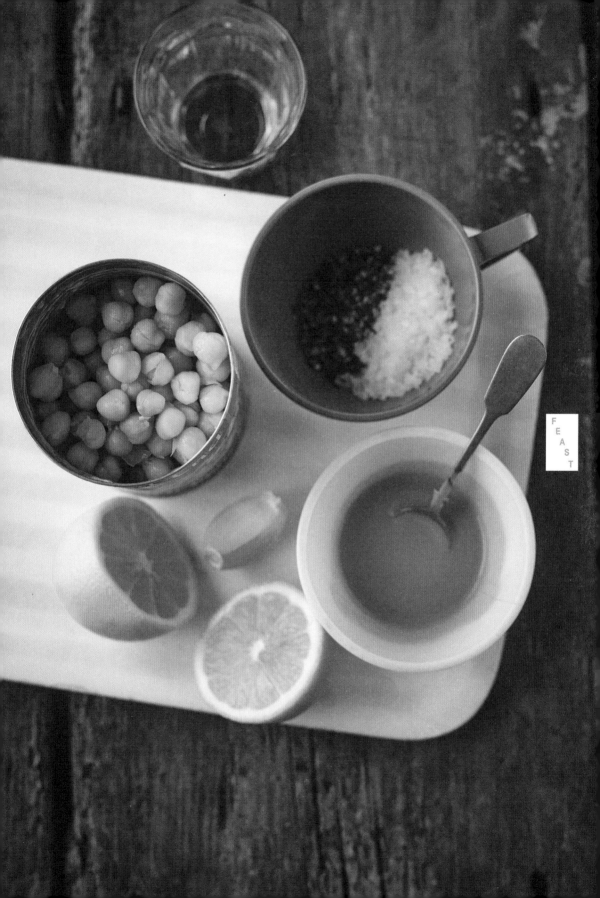

FEAST

... Beetroot and onion pickle/Golden amazing sauce/Kachumber/Walnut and basil pesto/Ginger and miso dressing/Pear Café seed blend/Marinated feta/Coconut and lime dressing/Tahini noodle dressing/Wild garlic oil/Brown butter

Important rainbow pickle/Pear Café Dressing/Pico de Gallo/Cajun spice blend/Zaatar ...

Sauces, Pickles and Dressings

Golden amazing sauce

37 kcal
per portion

If you're a fan of the hilarious American comedy show, *Parks and Recreation*, you'll get the Golden Amazing Sauce reference. If you love dressings that you can smother green veg/rice/fish – basically anything – in, you'll get the sauce. I've tried it on avocado on toast (well good), drizzled on spiced lentil soup (really great), poured over warm brown rice and topped with smoked trout and greens (really, really delicious) and don't see any reason why you shouldn't try it on all sorts of other things. It's also used in the Raw Rainbow Salad on page 64.

I calculated the recipe as 3 kcal for 1g, so measure it carefully on fast days and it can certainly be part of a fast-day meal. On feast days, use it with wild abandon!

Makes about 250ml (roughly 20 portions

—

60ml extra-virgin
    olive oil

25g tahini

50g tinned chickpeas,
    drained and rinsed

1 garlic clove, crushed

45ml fresh lemon juice

½ tsp turmeric

10g Marmite

Blitz all the ingredients together with 60ml cold water until completely smooth. That's it!

The sauce will keep well in a sealed jar in the fridge for a week or so – just give it a really good shake before you use it.

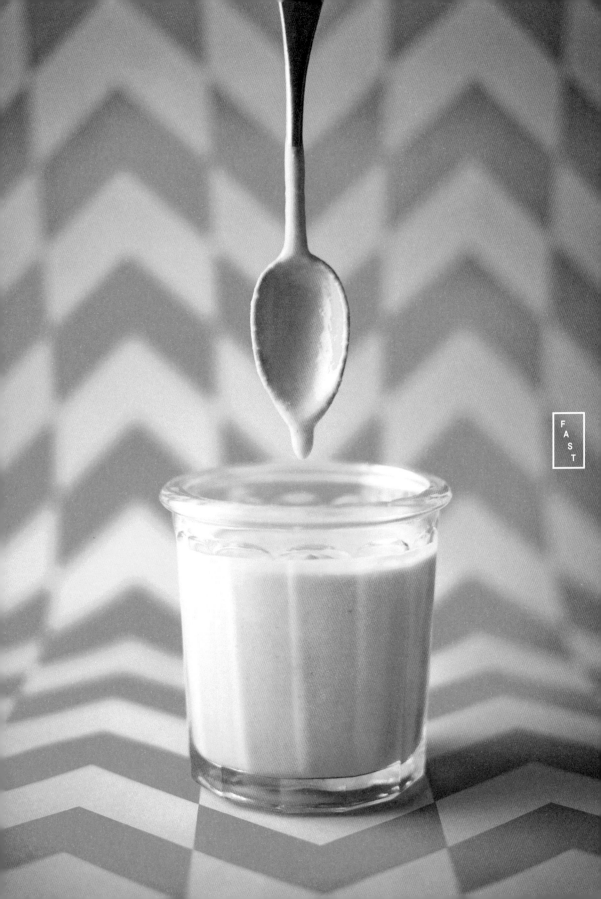

Beetroot and onion pickle

This pickle/salsa/salad is a great accompaniment to a dhal or a curry, and any leftovers can be popped in the fridge and used up over the next few days in salads, etc. I do, however, prefer it on the day it's made, when it's still really crunchy and tastes fresh.

**Makes 270g (about
5 portions at 54g each)**
—

130g white onions,
   finely diced

120g raw beetroot, any
   colour, finely diced
   or grated

1 tbsp flaked sea salt

30ml sherry vinegar

10g date syrup

handful of chopped coriander

Put the diced onions and beetroot in a colander and sprinkle with salt. Leave to stand for approximately 20 minutes.

Squeeze out as much liquid as possible.

Combine all the remaining ingredients in a bowl and tip in the vegetables. Stir well and serve.

F
A
S
T

Ginger and miso dressing

You can whip this dressing up in seconds. Its transforming powers know no bounds. I love it drizzled over green veg, and it is fantastic used as a noodle dressing. Make double or triple quantities and keep covered in the fridge for up to three days. It is a delicious accompaniment to the Marinated Tofu with Greens and Brown Rice recipe on page 146 and is also used in the Edamame, pea, miso and ginger salad on page 59.

Makes 1 portion
—

8g white miso paste

1 tbsp fresh lemon juice

¼ garlic clove, very
   finely grated

1cm piece of root
   ginger, peeled and
   very finely grated

1 tsp sesame oil

½ tsp honey

Put all the ingredients with ½ tablespoon boiling water in a jar, seal and shake like mad. The mixture should be a pourable consistency, like double cream. Add up to another ½ tablespoon boiling water if it is too thick.

Kachumber

10 kcal
per portion

This is the salad/salsa you get given in Indian restaurants in the traditional chutney tray, along with mango chutney and raita. It's the low-cal member of that crew, so gets in on the fast-day action. Best served on the day you make it, it will however keep for up to three days in the fridge.

I love this with the Chickpea Curry on page 100, but it's also great mixed with prawns and shredded little gem lettuce.

Makes 285g,
5 portions of 57g
—

¼ tsp cumin seeds

4g coriander leaves

5g finely chopped green chilli

5 mint leaves, roughly chopped

55g onion, finely diced

95g cucumber, finely diced

120g tomato, finely diced

2 tsp fresh lemon juice

flaked sea salt

Toast the cumin seeds in a small dry pan over a low heat, until aromatic. Remove and add to a bowl with the remaining ingredients. Mix well and leave to sit for 30 minutes before serving.

F
A
S
T

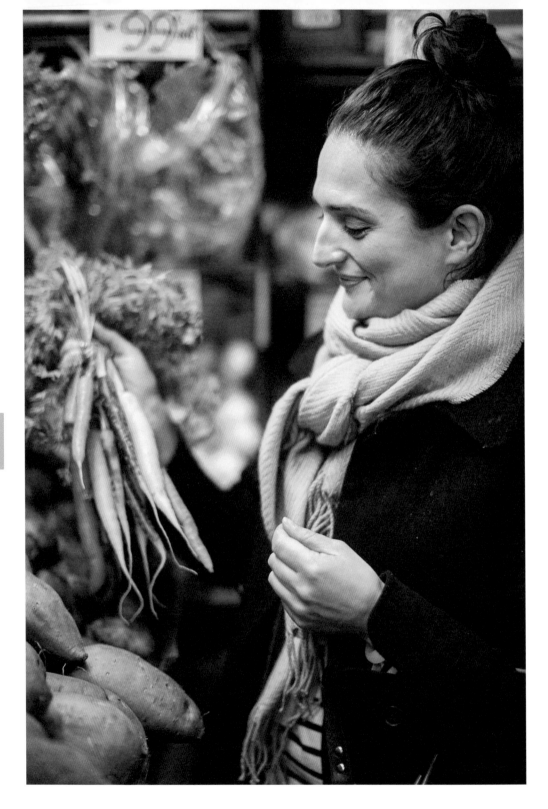

Impatient rainbow pickles

The instant pickle for the impatient cook. Basically, right up my strasse. I love pickles and I love the idea of filling jars with loads of preserved things, but I always want to eat them straight away.

In late spring or early summer you'll start to see big bunches of rainbow-coloured heritage carrots and radishes in farmers' markets and greengrocers. You can, of course, use any carrots or radishes for this, but the multicoloured ones will be extra pretty. Feel free to try pickling other vegetables using the same liquid recipe and method.

Especially good on tacos and alongside seared salmon, these pickles are great to have in the fridge as they will lend crunch and sweetness to loads of dishes.

Makes 2 x 500ml

—

2 bunches of radish (approximately 15–20 radishes), multicoloured if possible

8–10 small carrots, multi-coloured if possible

¼ red onion, thinly sliced

4–6 rainbow chard stalks, cut into batons, 5mm wide

3 tbsp roughly chopped pickled jalapeños

4 tbsp roughly chopped fresh coriander

2 big pinches of flaked sea salt

250ml white wine vinegar

250ml apple cider vinegar

120ml red wine vinegar

360g sugar

2 tsp coriander seeds, toasted and crushed

Using a mandoline or a very sharp knife, slice the radishes and carrots into 1–2mm thick slices. Put into a large bowl. Add the onion, chard, jalapeños, fresh coriander and salt.

Bring the vinegars, sugar and coriander seeds to a gentle boil in a medium pan and whisk over a medium heat until all the sugar has dissolved. Remove from the heat and leave to cool to room temperature.

Once cool, add the pickling liquid to the bowl with the vegetables, jalapeños, coriander and salt and combine well. Divide the veg mixture between two jars, pour over the pickling liquid, making sure all the veg is covered well. Alternatively, pour the whole lot into a Tupperware container.

Store in the fridge for at least 2 hours before eating, and up to 3 weeks. Occasionally make sure the veg is submerged in the liquid to prevent any oxidation. The beautiful colours will start to fade after a couple of days but the pickles will still taste amazing.

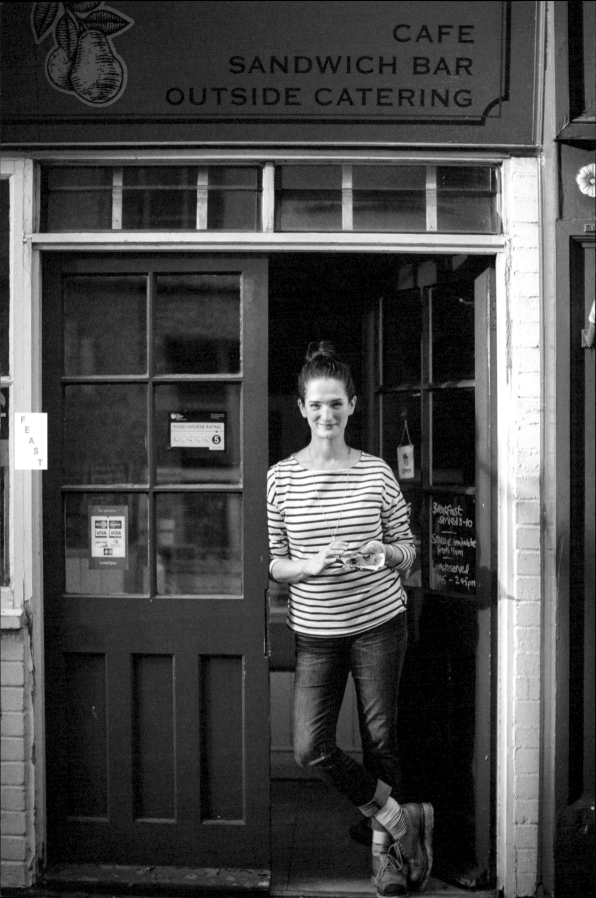

Pear Café Dressing

This is our 'house dressing' at the café. We've been making it for years. It is used in our salads and has become an integral component of some of our sandwiches – most notably, our Grandma's Egg and Onion on page 94. Honey, mustard and balsamic dressings are a bit 90s, aren't they? We don't care. This dressing is lush.

Makes about 230ml
—
150ml extra-virgin
   olive oil
50ml balsamic vinegar
1 tbsp wholegrain mustard
1 tbsp runny honey

Put everything into a clean jar, put the lid on and shake really hard. Taste and adjust to your personal preference by adding more of any of the ingredients. Keeps for at least 2 weeks in the fridge.

Pear Café seed blend

These seeds go into our salads and some of our sandwiches at the café – they feature in our Grandma's Egg and Onion (see page 94), where they bring their toasty nuttiness to the egg mayo and gherkin party.

At home, I keep a jar of these on hand and add them to the majority of my meals: egg dishes and avocado on toast at brunch and Buddha bowls. Salads are made infinitely better and more nutritious with a scattering of seeds. Be mindful on fast days, though, as the seeds are pretty calorific – add sparingly and, as always, weigh and measure out.

Multiply or divide the quantities as much as you like, as long as you keep the ratios roughly the same.

Makes about 100g
—
2 tbsp sesame seeds
2 tbsp pumpkin seeds
2 tbsp sunflower seeds
1 tbsp nigella seeds

Tip all the seeds into a dry frying pan and set over a medium heat. Toast for 8–10 minutes, shaking the pan to mix the seeds well and watching them like a hawk at all times. They'll burn easily.

As soon as the pumpkin seeds start to split slightly and the sesame seeds are golden brown, take off the heat. Let the seeds cool completely. Store in an airtight container, where they'll stay crunchy for weeks.

Cajun spice blend

1 kcal
per ¼ tsp

Use this spice blend in the Cajun Prawns (page 160), the Jambalaya-ish (page 162) and the Cajun Split Pea and Corn soup (page 110). Keep it on hand to add to the Lentil and Red Pepper Chilli (page 102) if you fancy it a bit punchier or add half a teaspoon to the Sweet Potato Wedges (page 145) to give them even more fire.

½ tsp smoked paprika

½ tsp cayenne pepper

½ tsp dried oregano

½ tsp dried thyme

½ tsp dried chilli flakes

In a bowl, mix the ingredients together. The spice blend will keep for XX, stored in an airtight jar.

Za'atar

8 kcal
per 1 tsp

F
A
S
T

Use this in the Lebanese-style Breakfast (page 38). It also makes a delicious addition to a chickpea and tomato salad or roast broccoli salad. Having a bowl of this and a bowl of argan or olive oil side by side makes a great bread dip, too. Take a chunk of bread, dip it into some oil and then into the za'atar. Ta-daa! Snack city.

Makes 150g

—

3 tbsp sesame seeds

2 tbsp dried thyme

3 tbsp ground sumac

1 tbsp flaked sea salt

1 tbsp ground cumin

Toast the sesame seeds in a small, dry pan over low heat until lightly golden. Remove from the heat and put in a small bowl with the thyme, sumac, salt and ground cumin. Keeps for ages in an airtight jar.

Tahini noodle dressing

Makes about 200ml

50g tahini

1 tbsp soy sauce

2 tbsp sesame oil

3 tbsp rice vinegar

2 tsp date syrup

3 garlic cloves, crushed

¼ tsp chipotle chilli flakes

1 tsp flaked sea salt

1.5cm piece root ginger,
    finely grated

Blitz all the ingredients with 1½ tablespoons of warm water in a food processor or blender, until fully combined.

Use to dress noodles while still warm.

The dressing will keep happily in the fridge in a lidded jar for up to 3 days.

Roasted red pepper sauce

Like a romesco sauce, this contains roasted peppers and almonds. It doesn't include bread, however, and the tahini and date syrup make it sweeter and creamier than its cousin.

Serves 6

55g blanched almonds

280g tomatoes, chopped

50g tahini

1 tsp sherry vinegar

1 tsp date syrup

2 tsp sweet smoked paprika

1 tsp flaked sea salt

freshly ground black pepper

For the roasted red peppers

4 red peppers, halved
    and deseeded

¼ red onion, roughly chopped

5 garlic cloves, peeled

2 tbsp olive oil

sea salt and freshly
    ground black pepper,
    for seasoning

Preheat the oven to 230°C/430°F/Gas mark 7½.

Put the peppers, chopped onion and garlic in a roasting tray. Pour over the olive oil and season with salt and pepper. Bake for about 20 minutes, until the peppers and onion are charred and blackened at the edges. Take out of the oven and set aside to cool.

Transfer the roasted veg to a food processor or blender and blitz to a purée. Set to one side while you prepare the almonds.

Clean and dry the food processor. Add the almonds and blitz until you have the texture of sand. Remove and set aside.

Put the remaining ingredients in the food processor and blitz to form a XX paste. Add the ground almonds and the puréed peppers, and briefly pulse. This sauce is best eaten on the day it's made, but keeps in the fridge for up to 3 days.

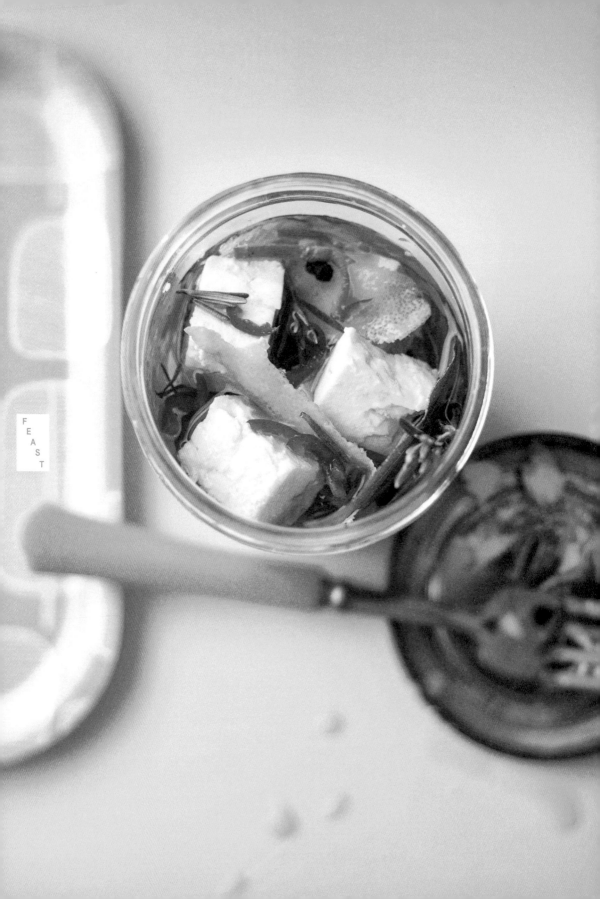

Marinated feta

Feta, once it's opened, does not last well. I like using it on fast days, as just a few grams adds a lovely cold creaminess and contrast to an otherwise crunchy salad or a hot bowl of chilli or stew.

Often I'm left with the majority of a packet to use up. If you're just cooking for one, this can mean you're eating feta meal after meal just to use it up quickly enough. If you marinate the leftover feta using this method, you extend its life for up to three weeks.

This recipe uses a whole block of feta, but make tweaks to the flavourings if you have more or less. If you're preserving more than one block, you'll need to add extra oil to ensure that the cheese is totally covered. This is vital and is the only thing that stops the cheese going off.

You could, of course, go and specifically buy feta, but that kind of destroys the point of preserving leftovers. That reminds me of my mum asking my Great Grandpa Aubrey for his excellent chopped liver recipe and starting by asking him how many chicken livers she needed. 'How many have you got?!' came his reply.

Makes 200g
—

1 x 200g packet feta, cut into strips or cubed

2 rosemary sprigs

½ red chilli, finely sliced

2 strips lemon zest

4 black peppercorns

1 bay leaf

olive oil, about 250ml or enough to cover

Put the feta into a shallow plastic tub (a takeaway container is perfect) or a Kilner jar.

Add the remaining ingredients and pour over enough olive oil to cover everything completely. Store in the fridge, where it will keep for up to 3 weeks.

Variation

For a cheaper and lower-calorie version, you can also preserve feta in salt water by dissolving 100g of flaked sea salt 1 litre of water. Bring to the boil and then allow to cool. This method will preserve the cheese for up to 3 weeks.

FEAST

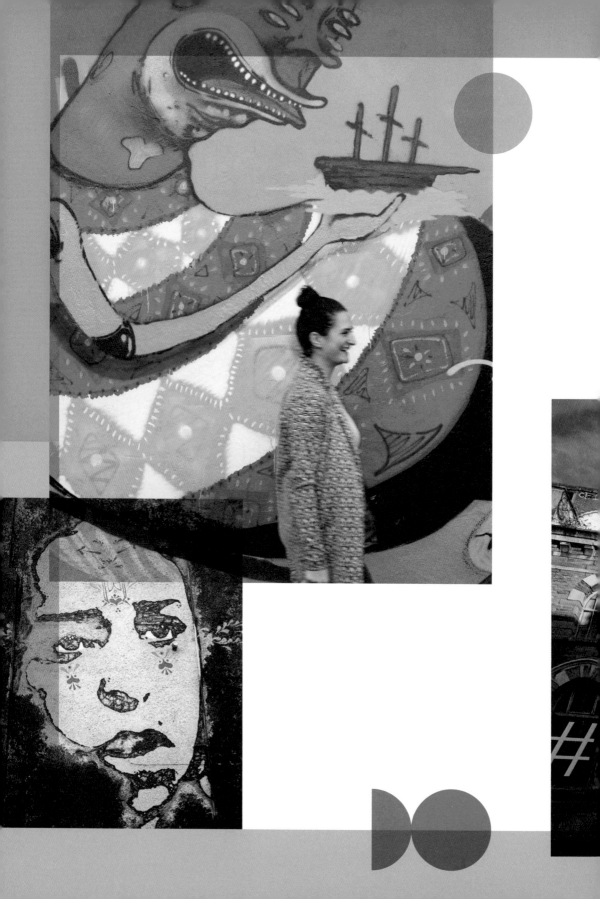

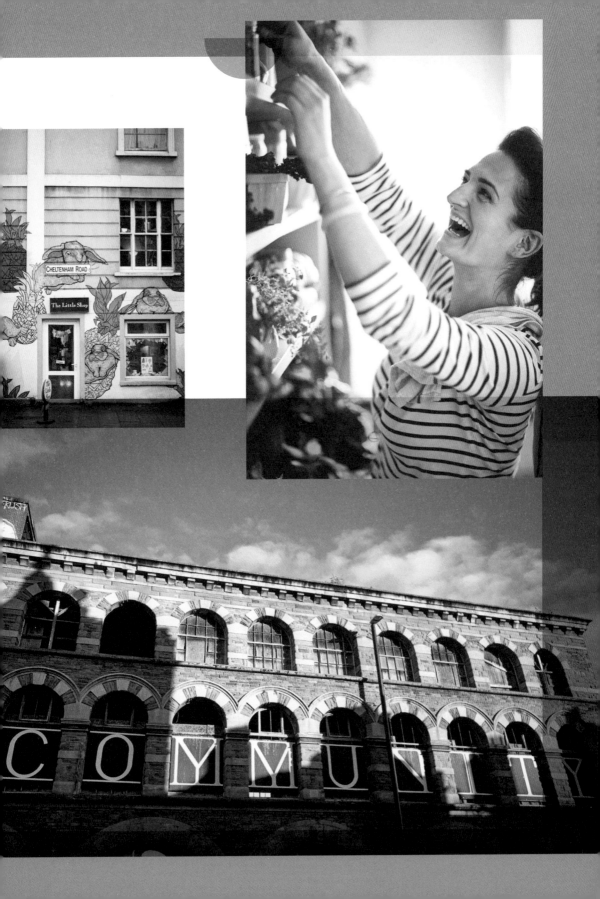

My secret weapon brown butter

This is my mate chef Tom Griffith's method for making brown butter. Once you've made brown butter it will keep in the fridge for up to two weeks. I like to make the full quantity on the day I'm having a dinner party, use it on the Seared Scallops on page 182 and the Roasted Cauliflower Meunière on page 195, then use it to fry eggs for breakfast the next day. See also the other suggestions below for using up the leftovers —although, as my mate Ed (@rocketandsquash) Smith said, 'I've never had leftover brown butter'.

Makes 200g

250g unsalted butter,
    cut into cubes

small handful of thyme sprigs

1 shallot, finely diced

¼ tsp sea salt

½ tsp freshly ground
    black pepper

juice of 1 lemon

In a small saucepan, add the butter, thyme, shallot and salt. Heat over a low heat for approximately 15 minutes, stirring constantly, until the butter is brown and small nutty.

Remove from the heat, pour the browned butter into a cold pan and set aside for 1 minute, then whisk in the lemon juice.

Leave to cool to room temperature, strain into a bowl and keep in the fridge, covered, ready to use whenever you like over the next couple of weeks.

Uses for leftover brown butter

Use it in the Pumpkin and Sage Soup on page 118.

Heat up a spoonful in a pan, add a few sage leaves and cook until crispy. Pour over a plate of gnocchi and roasted cubes of pumpkin.

Roast new potatoes, radishes and fennel in a little seasoned olive oil. Melt some brown butter, whisk in a little grain mustard and a little maple syrup and toss the cooked veg in it. Garnish with soft herbs such as parsley, mint or dill.

Use it to pan-fry a fillet of sea bream or sea bass.

Finish a risotto with a spoonful of it.

Toss asparagus spears in it and top with a poached egg.

Poach salted hake slowly in brown butter and flake it into a salad of little gem lettuce, roast tomatoes and aioli.

Pico de Gallo
(fresh tomato salsa)

3 kcal
per tbsp

This fast-day-friendly fresh tomato salsa is true to the classic recipe. It just happens to be very low in calories. Use as a dip with celery sticks or leaves of little gem, or top your chilli with a spoonful to add a great fresh crunch. I love it on a feast day, too, on my brunch plate, with the Root Veg and Halloumi Fritters (page 137) and a poached egg.

200g tomatoes, finely diced

80g onions, finely diced

40g pickled jalapeños, drained and finely diced

50g coriander, finely chopped (including stalks)

2 tbsp fresh lime juice

2 tsp white wine vinegar

1 tsp dried oregano

flaked sea salt and freshly ground black pepper

Put all the chopped vegetables and coriander in a bowl. Add the lime juice, vinegar and dried oregano. Mix well and season to taste.

F
A
S
T

Coconut and lime dressing

125ml coconut milk

2 tbsp soy sauce

zest of 1 lime, finely grated

2 tbsp lime juice

Simply blitz all the ingredients in a food processor or blender until thoroughly blended.

Walnut and basil pesto

Serves 2-4

50g walnuts

1 large handful of basil leaves

25g Parmesan, roughly chopped

¼ garlic clove, roughly chopped

3 tbsp olive oil, plus extra if needed

flaked sea salt and freshly ground black pepper

Toast the walnuts in a small, dry pan over a medium-low heat until nutty and slightly browned. Take off the heat and put in a mini food processor along with the remaining ingredients. Blitz until smooth, adding more olive oil if you want to thin out the pesto.

Alternative pestos

Kale or chard – substitute a handful of raw kale for the basil and replace the walnuts with pistachios.

Pea shoots or rocket – use up the last of a bag by whizzing them up into a pesto.

Sunflower seeds also make a good pesto.

Wild garlic oil

I hesitated about including this recipe, as wild garlic is not available to everyone. Even if you are near a patch, it's only around for a few weeks each year. However, each year I pick some and use it non-stop, while I can, and then mourn its loss once it's all gone. This year, I found a way of preserving it. Months later, as I write this, it's still in my fridge and still bright green. So every year from now onwards I'm going to keep that pungent, vibrant, garlicky green in my life a little longer than nature decrees.

Makes 250ml

2 really big handfuls of wild garlic
200ml olive oil or rapeseed oil

Rinse the wild garlic well and trim off any brown bits.

Bring a pan of water to the boil and add the wild garlic. Blanch for 5 seconds, then immediately use tongs to pull them out. Drain, refresh under cold water, then plunge into a bowl of iced water. Allow to drain.

Use your hands to squeeze as much water out as possible and put on a clean (but not precious) tea towel – it'll get stained bright green. Squeeze dry.

Chop the clump of squeezed leaves up roughly by running over it in all directions with a sharp knife.

Blitz in a blender or food processor with the olive or rapeseed oil. Keep adding more oil until it's as thin as you want it.

Pour through a fine sieve into a sterilised jar and keep in the fridge for up to 3 months.

FEAST

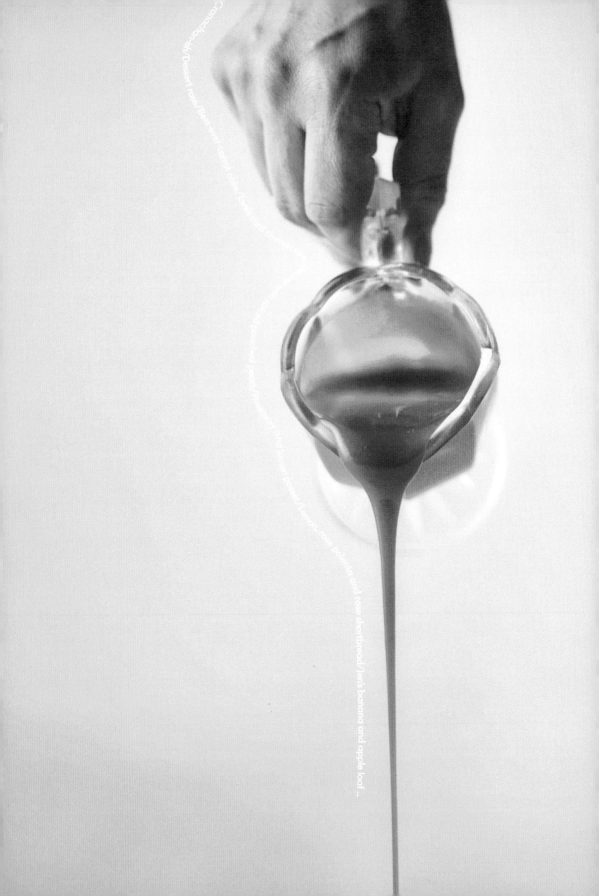

Puddings and Cakes

Lemon, polenta and rose shortbread

I made these pretty, crumbly, delicious biscuits for my mate Millie's baby shower. We did a massive brunch spread with huge piles of smoked salmon bagels fresh from Brick Lane, towers of chocolate brownies, fresh berries, frittata and Greek yoghurt swirled with date syrup and topped with pumpkin seeds. I roasted some rhubarb with cinnamon and served these little shortbreads on the side.

Once you make the dough and roll it, you can freeze it, then defrost, slice and bake when you want to serve your shortbread.

Makes about 25
—

100g unsalted butter, cold, cut into 1cm cubes

zest and juice of ¼ lemon

50g golden caster sugar

2 tbsp dried edible rose petals

100g plain flour, plus extra for dusting

100g polenta

Rub the butter, lemon zest, sugar, rose petals, flour and polenta together until they start to form a stiff dough. Add the lemon juice and knead into a rough ball. Dust the work surface with a little flour and roll the dough out into a long sausage shape, approximately 2.5cm in diameter. Wrap in cling film and chill in the fridge for 1 hour (or at this point you can freeze the dough, if you like – see above).

Preheat the oven to 150°C/300°F/Gas mark 2. Line a baking tray (or two) with baking parchment. Cut the sausage into 5mm thick slices. Lay the slices out on the prepared tray, leaving a space of about 2.5cm between each one – the biscuits will spread a little during baking.

Bake for 15 minutes, until the shortbread are 'blonde' with just a hint of tan. Take out of the oven and leave them on the baking tray, without moving them, for 5 minutes. Then carefully, using a palette knife, move them onto a wire rack to cool completely. As with all biscuits, these will crisp up once cooled. They keep well in an airtight tin for a few days.

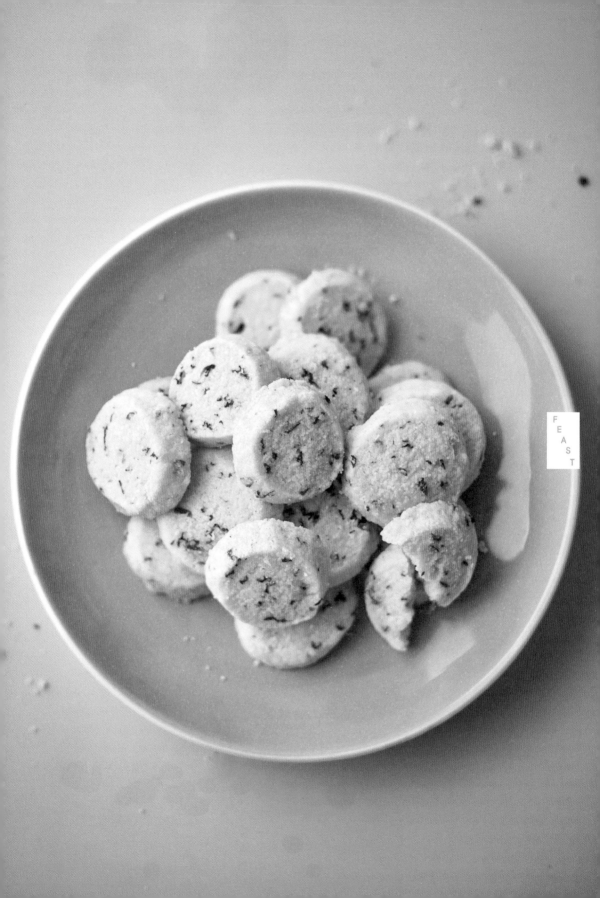
FEAST

Banana and oat bars

These bars are wheat free, vegan and sugar free, but still taste fantastic. Weird, huh?

I've added toasted hazelnuts, dried cranberries and chunks of chocolate to the mix in the past. All worked very well. Have a play about.

Makes 12

—

90ml olive oil, plus
    extra for greasing
75g raisins
100ml apple juice
200g jumbo oats
60g ground almonds
30g desiccated coconut
2 large pinches of sea salt
4 very ripe bananas
¼ tsp vanilla extract

Preheat the oven to 180°C/350°F/Gas mark 4. Grease a 20cm square, 5cm deep tin with a little olive oil.

Put the raisins in a small bowl and pour the apple juice over. Set aside for 30 minutes for the raisins to soak up the juice.

In a separate bowl, combine the oats with the ground almonds, coconut and salt.

In a food processor or using a stick blender, whizz the bananas, vanilla and olive oil into a smoothish paste, leaving some small chunks of banana. Combine the oat mix with the banana mixture and add the soaked raisins, along with the juice. Mix well.

Pour into the greased tin, smooth over the surface and bake for about 25 minutes, until firm and light brown. If it looks like it's getting too brown, cover loosely with foil.

Leave to cool in the tin for 10 minutes, then transfer to a wire rack to cool completely before cutting into 12 slices.

These bars keep very well in an airtight tin for up to 5 days.

F
E
A
S
T

Best-ever carrot cake

This is a huge cake. It'll serve ten massive slices. Unlike a sponge cake, carrot cake keeps well because it's so moist, making it perfect for a celebration if you need to have a cake baked in advance. Once it's totally cool, wrap the cake tightly in a few layers of cling film and keep it in an airtight tin or Tupperware container. Make the icing up to a day in advance, keep it in the fridge and ice the cake just before you want to serve it.

Serves 10–12
——

300g self-raising flour

225g plain flour

1 tsp bicarbonate of soda

2½ tsp ground cinnamon

2½ tsp ground nutmeg

220g light muscovado sugar
    or soft light brown sugar

220g golden caster sugar

300g grated carrot

100g sultanas

100g walnuts, roughly
    chopped

310ml vegetable oil

5 eggs, lightly beaten

300g soured cream

2 tsp vanilla extract

For the icing

250g cream cheese, at
    room temperature

750g icing sugar, sifted

500g unsalted
    butter, at room
    temperature

seeds from 1 vanilla pod

Preheat the oven to 180°C/350°F/Gas mark 4. Grease and line a 25cm round cake tin with baking parchment.

Sift the flours, bicarbonate of soda and spices into a large bowl. Add the sugars, carrot, sultanas and walnuts and stir to combine.

In a separate bowl, whisk the oil, eggs, soured cream and vanilla until smooth.

Add the wet ingredients to the dry ingredients and stir until just combined.

Pour into the tin, smoothing over the top and bake in the centre of the oven for 2 hours, or until a skewer inserted into the centre of the cake comes out clean.

Remove from the oven and leave to cool in the tin for 20 minutes. Turn out onto a wire rack to cool completely.

Make the icing by mixing all the ingredients in a food processor until fully combined.

When you're ready to serve the cake, use a bread knife to carefully split it in half using small see-saw motions.

Spread a third of the icing over the bottom half of the cake and sandwich with the top. Ice the top in thick swirls and leave the sides naked.

Serve with a big satisfied smile. This is a wicked cake.

F
E
A
S
T

Ewe's curd cheesecake mousse
with spiced poached pears

I very, very rarely make anything that takes me longer than half an hour to make. I'm too impatient. But sometimes you've just gotta bust out the big guns and do something extra special. If you can break a long recipe down into sections that you can do over a few days, it spreads the workload and stops it feeling like a slog. This is a dessert we served up at our supper club a few times. As the seasons changed, we used different fruits and tried a variety of biscuit-type accompaniments. It's a (delicious) blank canvas that happily sits alongside all sorts of other flavours. Once it's made, it can sit in the fridge for up to four days and can simply be scooped into fancy quenelles once you're ready to serve. In restaurants, desserts are often designed to incorporate ready-made elements like this so that the wait time is minimised. You then compile all the ready and waiting elements in a matter of moments.

    The clever technique for the mousse comes from Scottish chef Tom Kitchin. You're basically making a cheesecake (without a base), then baking it before blitzing it all up again and chilling it. Weird, original and wonderful. He uses crowdie, which is a Scottish cream cheese, but I find that ewe's curd works really well, as does a mild, rindless goat's cheese or mascarpone.

Serves 4–6
—

450g ewe's curd (or 125g rindless soft goat's cheese, 75g feta and 250g mascarpone)

125g caster sugar

1¼ tbsp plain flour

1 tbsp vanilla extract, or the seeds from 1 vanilla pod

finely grated zest of 1 lemon

1 whole egg, plus 1 egg yolk

Fatty's Salted Caramel Sauce, warmed, to serve (see page 246)

Preheat the oven to 150°C/300°F/Gas mark 2.

Blitz the cheese, sugar, flour, vanilla and lemon zest in a blender or food processor until totally smooth. In a jug, mix the egg and egg yolk together, then pour into the blender with the cheese mixture and blend until smooth.

Pour into a 23cm baking dish and cover tightly with foil. Bake for 35–40 minutes until set. Remove and allow to cool for 30 minutes. Transfer the mixture to a blender and blitz until completely smooth. Leave to set in the fridge for at least 1 hour.

You can serve the cheesecake once it's set and cold in the fridge, or keep it in the fridge, covered, for up to 4 days.

To make the spiced pears, peel them, leaving the stalks on. Cut a slice off the base of each pear that so they stand upright. Set aside.

For the spiced poached pears

4 pears
juice of 1 lemon
600ml dessert wine
250g caster sugar
1 bay leaf
2 peppercorns
1 cinnamon stick
2 star anise
1 vanilla pod
1 clove

Put the remaining ingredients, along with 200ml water, in a pan. Bring to the boil, reduce the heat, then simmer for 10 minutes until the sugar dissolves. Add the pears (standing them upright) and simmer, covered, for 5 minutes. Turn the heat off and let the pears cool down in the spiced liquid. Carefully cut the pears in half and lay them in a Tupperware container. Pour the liquid over them and leave to stand for 1 hour.

Serve two pear halves per person, with some of the cheesecake mousse and the salted caramel sauce, slightly warmed, in a small jug on the side.

FEAST

Fatty's salted caramel sauce

This recipe belongs to my friend Chloe Timms, who set up her own company making salted caramels. She called it Fatties Bakery, and although she is anything but, we all know her as Fatty.

Created by Chloe especially for this book, the result is slightly sharper than her regular salted caramel sauce. The addition of lemon juice balances the sweetness of the cheesecake mousse and the poached pears (see page 244), but it also means that it goes brilliantly with vanilla ice cream or even as a layer on top of the Chocolate and PX Pots on page 253.

Thank you, Fatty!

Makes just over 200g

—

85g double cream

1 tsp vanilla extract

a good pinch of sea salt

125g caster sugar

1 tbsp glucose syrup

30g slightly salted
    butter, cubed

1 tsp lemon juice

Begin by measuring the cream, vanilla and salt into a small, heavy-based saucepan. Set over a gentle heat, allowing it to warm but not boil, then remove from the heat, cover and keep warm.

Combine the caster sugar, glucose syrup and 2 tablespoons of water in a clean, heavy-based pan. Put the pan over a medium-low heat and cook, without mixing, gently to dissolve the sugar. (Use a brush dipped in warm water to clean the insides of the pan if sugar crystals start to form.) Continue to heat the sugar until it is the colour of a copper penny and begins to smoke. Be patient and keep an eagle eye on it. If needed, give it a swirl every now and then to ensure even caramelisation.

Once deep and smoky, immediately remove the pan from the heat and whisk in the warm cream mixture. Watch out for steam burn!

Stir in the cubed butter and lemon juice.

Serve immediately in a jug, or let it cool to room temperature and then store in the fridge, where it will last for at least 2 weeks. Warm gently before serving.

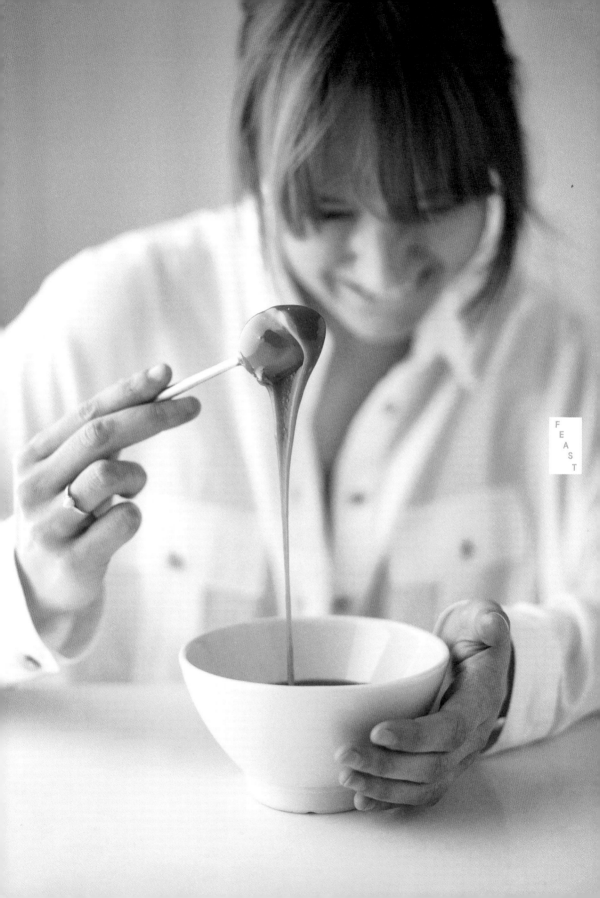

Rosemary and lemon posset with Italian meringue

This dessert is comprised of three elements – a nutty crumble base, a creamy rosemary infused lemon posset and topped off with browned Italian meringue. It's not a quick recipe, but it's totally worth it. As you plunge your teaspoon into the glass, you hit greater and greater resistance as you move through the layers of soft meringue, dense, smooth posset and finally the crumbly base. It's heavenly and I've never met a person who didn't love this dish. A proper special-occasion crowd-pleaser.

The first time we tried to make Italian meringue we used a food processor with an egg-whipping attachment. Because the heat couldn't escape out of the closed top, it went really wrong. You really need a standmixer to make Italian meringue, or a large bowl and an electric whisk.

Serves 4–6, depending on serving glass size

—

For the crumble base
100g plain flour
50g dark brown sugar
25g golden syrup
pinch of sea salt
75g unsalted butter, at room temperature
50g jumbo or porridge oats
20g chopped hazelnuts

Preheat the oven to 180°C/350°F/Gas mark 4, and line a baking tray with baking parchment.

Place the flour, sugar, golden syrup, salt and soft butter in a bowl. Use your fingertips to rub the butter into the flour, until you have the consistency of coarse breadcrumbs. Add the oats and chopped hazelnuts and mix well. Transfer the crumble mixture to the lined baking tray, even out the top and bake for 20 minutes, stirring once during the cooking time.

Remove and allow to cool, then break up any extra-large chunks. Put a tablespoon of the crumble into each serving glass.

To make the posset, put the cream, sugar and rosemary in a large saucepan, over a low heat, and gently bring to the boil. Boil for exactly 3 minutes, then take off the heat and allow to cool.

Add the lemon zest and juice. Whisk well. Strain the mixture through a fine sieve into a jug, then carefully pour into the serving glasses containing the crumble. Refrigerate for 3 hours, until set.

For the Italian meringue, wash your standmixer bowl with very hot, soapy water and dry with a scrupulously clean tea towel. If there's any grease in your bowl, the egg whites won't whisk up.

For the rosemary-infused posset

400ml double cream

100g caster sugar

1 rosemary sprig, leaves picked and chopped

grated zest and juice of 1 lemon

For the Italian meringue

120g egg whites (free-range liquid egg whites are available in a carton from the supermarket, or if using whole eggs, use about 4 large eggs and separate the yolks from the whites very carefully)

300g caster sugar

You'll also need

an electric mixer (preferably a standmixer)

a sugar thermometer

2 x disposable piping bags

a 2.5cm round nozzle

a blowtorch

Now, put your egg whites into the bowl of your standmixer (you could also do this with electric whisks).

In a small saucepan, dissolve the sugar in 120ml water over a low heat, stirring until the sugar has dissolved. Once the sugar has dissolved, turn the heat up to medium and allow the syrup to come to the boil. Heat to 121°C/250°F.

Meanwhile, as soon as the temperature reaches 115°C/240°F, start whisking the egg whites in your standmixer, until they start to foam on the surface.

Still whisking, take the sugar syrup off the heat and pour it over the egg whites, in a thin stream. Be careful not to let the syrup touch the beaters. Continue to whisk until the eggs are lukewarm. The end result should be very stiff, smooth and satiny.

At this point, you can fill a disposable piping bag with the mixture and leave it in the fridge until you're ready to continue. You could even do this the day before.

Snip the end off your piping bag and put it inside another bag, fitted with a wide, round nozzle. Pipe some Italian meringue on top of your (now set) lemon posset. Decorate with whatever fetching meringue shape you feel is appropriate. Using a blowtorch, lightly brown the meringue.

And then eat it.

F
E
A
S
T

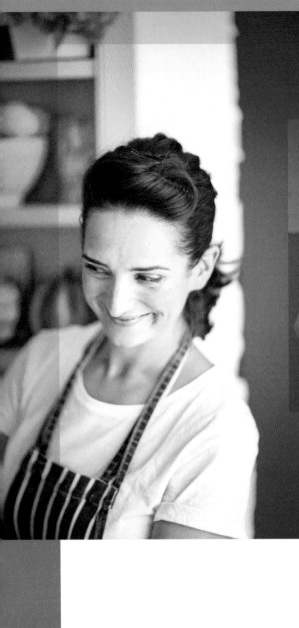
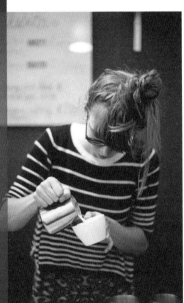
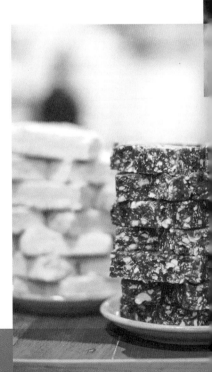
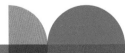

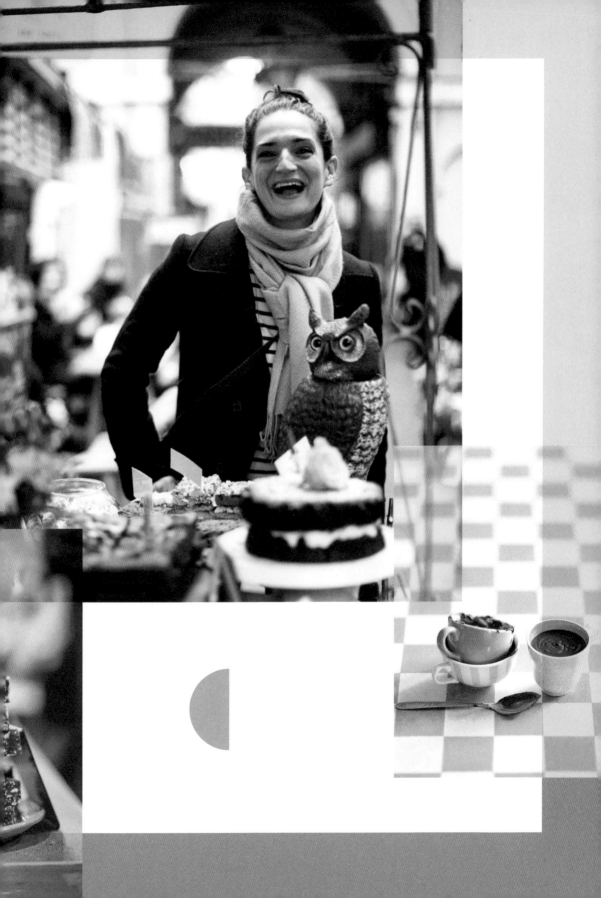

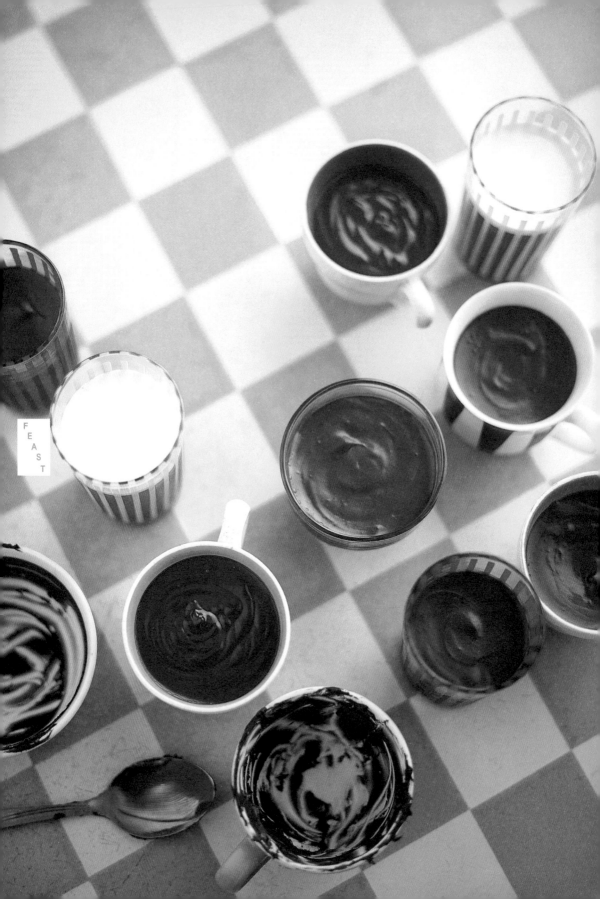

Chocolate and PX pots with cream

Serve each one in a little glass with a layer of cold cream, looking like a mini pint of Guinness. They're a great dinner-party dessert that can be made up to 3 days in advance and then served with no extra work. They're as rich as truffles, so don't worry that they look small. Any bigger and your guests will feel a bit pukey.

'PX' is shorthand for Pedro Ximénez – a gorgeously rich, sweet sherry made with sun-dried Pedro Ximénez grapes.

You can also swap the sherry for brandy. I'd leave out the cinnamon if you do. Or for a Mexican-style chocolate pot, add a little golden tequila, cinnamon and chilli.

Makes 6 small espresso-sized portions

—

150ml double cream, plus a little extra cold cream for serving (optional)

90ml full-cream milk

1 tbsp PX (Pedro Ximénez) sherry

175g good-quality dark chocolate, at least 75% cocoa solids (the best you can afford, as it really makes a difference), very finely chopped

¼ tsp vanilla essence

½ tsp ground cinnamon

50g caster sugar

1 egg

Heat the cream, milk and sherry in a saucepan over a medium heat until gently simmering. Add the chocolate and stir well, continuously, for about 5 minutes, until it has completely melted into the mixture. Turn the heat down to very low. Add the vanilla, cinnamon and sugar and cook for 3 minutes, stirring continuously and being careful to let the mixture boil, until all the sugar has dissolved.

Remove the pan from the heat and let cool for 10 minutes. Whisk in the egg.

Carefully pour the mixture between six glasses, giving them a tap on the table to get rid of any air bubbles. Chill for 4 hours, until set.

When you're ready to serve, pour a thin layer (2–5mm) of cold cream on top, if you like.

Cranachan-ish

Cranachan is a traditional Scottish dish made with piles of whipped cream, oats, whisky, honey and fresh raspberries. I've swapped the double cream for yoghurt and just used a small amount of toasted oats as a garnish. There's also a bigger ratio of raspberries than is traditional. That's why it's Cranachan-ish. Not the real deal, but delicious all the same.

Serves 1

¼ tsp whisky
50g 0% Greek yoghurt
5g jumbo oats
70g raspberries
¼ tsp date syrup

Mix the whisky with the yoghurt.

Toast the oats in a small, dry frying pan over a medium heat.

Layer up the raspberries and the yoghurt in small glasses or bowls, then drizzle with the syrup and sprinkle the toasted oats on top.

F
A
S
T

Strawberry, lime and basil granita

50 kcal
per portion

Most granita recipes use refined white sugar, but I wanted to experiment with an alternative. Date syrup is sweet, yes, but also amazingly deeply fruity. Read the whole recipe through before starting and make it when you are planning to be in for the whole of the evening, so that you can be near your freezer for about four or five hours.

Serves 1

—

400g ripe strawberries, hulled and roughly chopped

4 tbsp lime juice

15 basil leaves

90g date syrup

Put all the ingredients into a food processor or blender, along with 100ml water, and blitz until smooth.

Pour the mixture into a shallow dish with a decent-sized surface area, ideally about 20cm square.

Place in the freezer (you don't need to cover it) for a couple of hours until ice crystals start to form around the edges.

Use a fork to break the ice up and give the whole thing a good stir, scraping the frozen bits back into the mixture.

Place back in the freezer. Repeat this every hour or so over a period of 4–5 hours until the granita is frozen and fluffy.

Use a fork to scrape the surface up and then spoon the scrapings into small glasses.

The granita can be stored in the freezer, covered, until you want to serve more. If you're not on a fast day, liqueurs poured over the granita make for a refreshing end to a meal. A dash of Stellacello Pompelmo over this also works brilliantly.

F
A
S
T

Yoghurt, meringue and fruit

The real queen of yoghurt, meringue and fruit dishes is the Dessert Rose opposite, but there are lots of other combos that are quicker, a little less fancy and need fewer ingredients. Play around. This is a fast-day staple you'll be pleased you discovered.

Obviously weigh/measure and add everything into your calorie counter app carefully. Optional extras such as date syrup, mint, nuts and seeds are welcome additions. Buy mini meringues and check the label carefully.

natural yoghurt or 0% Greek yoghurt (check the label and use your calorie counter app to calculate how many calories)

fruit of your choice (see the Fruity Breakfast Options, page 46 for ideas)

mini meringue

optional extras of choice

Put the yoghurt into the bottom of a small glass and top with your fruit. Crumble over a mini meringue and top with optional extras, if using.

86 kcal

70g Greek yoghurt
30g mango
25g blueberries
1 mini meringue

90 kcal

60g 0% Greek yoghurt
50g blackberries
40g apple
1 mini meringue
1 mint sprig

74 kcal

70g 0% Greek yoghurt
50g strawberries
1 mini meringue

67 kcal

60g 0% Greek yoghurt
30g raspberries
1 mini meringue
1g desiccated coconut
1 mint sprig

90 kcal

65g 0% Greek yoghurt
60g pear
1 mini meringue
4g date syrup

87 kcal

70g 0% Greek yoghurt
50g blood orange
25g blueberries
1 mini meringue

76 kcal

60g natural yoghurt
65g pink grapefruit
1 mini meringue

80 kcal

60g natural yoghurt
40g peach, sliced
30g passion fruit flesh
1 mini meringue

Dessert rose

People are surprised to hear I regularly have a pudding on fast days. It's often a variation on this dish and there are countless ways you can adapt the basic recipe (see opposite page).

The date nectar and dried rose petals came from a local shop, but both can be purchased online. The date nectar (also called date syrup) adds a special flavour, but if you can't find it, maple syrup or dark agave nectar make good substitutes. Their calorie count is fairly similar, but always check the label and use an app like MyFitnessPal to calculate the calories.

Feel free to use different fruit or seed combos as opposite.

Makes 1 portion
—

3g unsalted pistachios

3g pumpkin seeds

50g low-fat natural plain yoghurt

25g raspberries

25g blueberries

1 mini meringue

3g date syrup

1 tsp dried edible rose petals

Gently toast the pistachios and pumpkin seeds in a small, dry frying pan over a low heat, until they brown. Remove from the heat and tip onto a chopping board to cool.

Spoon the yoghurt into the centre of a small bowl or deep plate.

Add the berries and then crumble over the meringue.

Roughly chop the nuts and seeds.

Drizzle the date syrup over the meringue and sprinkle with the rose petals, nuts and seeds.

F
A
S
T

Tropical treat yoghurt

This is a feast-day version of what I usually make on fast days for pudding. Mascarpone mixed with natural yoghurt was a discovery I only made when I had a little bit of each to use up. It's absolutely gorgeous but feel free to substitute Greek yoghurt for both. Go full-on tropical and replace the peach with banana if you like.

Serves 2
—

2 tsp pumpkin seeds

a small handful of
    coconut flakes

160g plain natural yoghurt

80g mascarpone

160g peach (1 large or
    2 small)

2 tsp date syrup

1 passion fruit

Toast the pumpkin seeds in a dry pan over a medium-low heat until they start to pop. Remove and cool. Toast the coconut flakes in the same pan until they start to turn golden brown. Remove and cool.

Mix the yoghurt and the mascarpone in a bowl until smooth.

Divide this mixture between bowls.

Cut the peach into wedges and divide between the bowls. Drizzle over the date syrup and add the seeds of half a passion fruit to each bowl.

Sprinkle with the toasted seeds and coconut flakes, then serve.

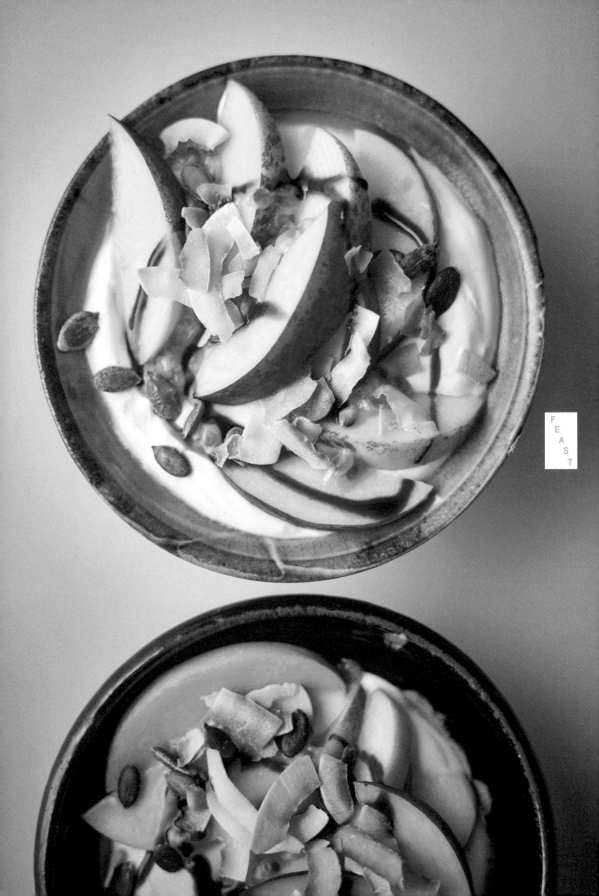

FEAST

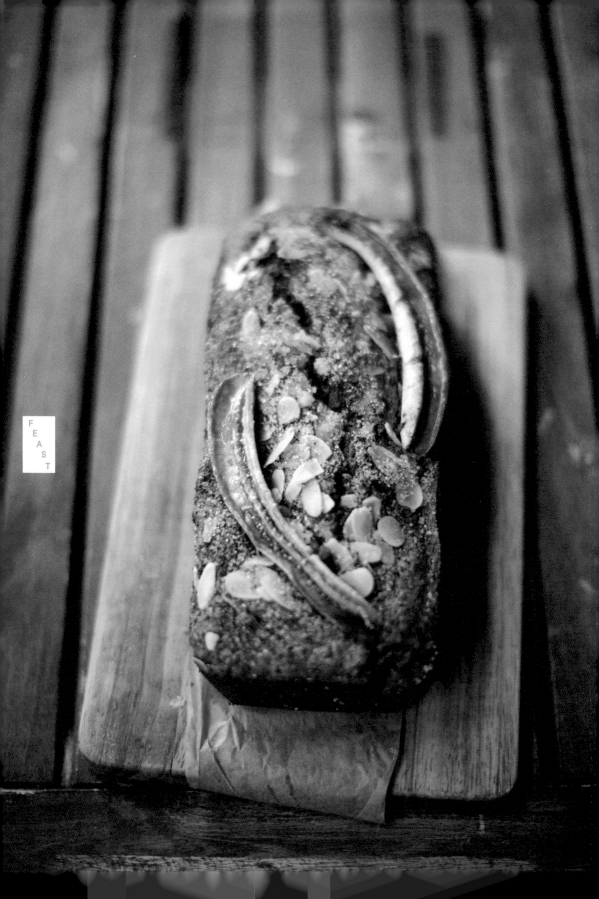

Jen's banana and apple loaf

People are very particular about their bananas. Once the smallest of brown patches appears, we watch as café customers reject them, searching through the pile in the fruit bowl for the 'perfect specimen'. So we have to find a way to use up these 'rejects', and, of course, banana loaf is the obvious answer. We sell loads of it at the café and have spent years experimenting with toppings and additions, such as nuts, to the cake mix. What follows is the result of much perfecting and adjusting, and it was café babe Jen who finally put the cherry (banana) on the top and created its great decorative topping.

It keeps well (as long as it's well wrapped up) and is mega moist. A winner of a cake.

Makes 1 loaf
(approximately 10 slices)
—

For the cake
150g salted butter
270g light brown
    muscovado sugar
2 eggs
200g peeled, very ripe
    bananas, mashed
    until really smooth
280g plain flour, plus
    plus 10g for dusting
1 tsp baking powder
1 tsp bicarbonate of soda
1 tsp ground cinnamon
1 tsp ground ginger
60g eating apple,
    chopped into
    1cm cubes

For the first topping
15g demerara sugar
15g pumpkin seeds

For the second topping
1 whole ripe banana
10g desiccated coconut
5g demerara sugar

Preheat the oven to 170°C/325°F/Gas mark 3.

Melt the butter in a small saucepan.

Whisk the sugar and eggs together until totally combined, then switch to a rubber spatula and blend in the mashed banana. Add the flour, baking powder, bicarbonate of soda, spices and apple and mix well.

Tip nearly all of the melted butter into the bowl, then rest the buttery pan upside down in a 23cm x 13cm loaf tin so that the excess butter can drip in.

Mix the butter into the cake mixture until totally incorporated and uniform in colour.

Use kitchen paper to spread the melted butter over the base and inner sides of the tin, then dust with the additional flour.

Pour the mixture into the tin and smooth out the surface. Sprinkle the demerara sugar and the pumpkin seeds for the first topping on the top.

Bake for an initial 30 minutes. Meanwhile, prepare the second topping. Peel and cut the banana in half, lengthways. When the 30 minutes is up, take the loaf out of the oven and, working quickly, lay the banana on top in a yin-yang formation. Next, sprinkle the coconut in the gaps around the banana and top with the demerara sugar. Bake for a further 30 minutes or until a skewer inserted into the centre of the cake comes out clean.

Remove from the oven and leave to cool in the tin for 30 minutes before carefully turning out onto a wire rack to cool completely.

FEAST

Sample
Fast Day
Menus

total calorie count

	Breakfast	Lunch	Dinner	Drinks	Snacks
487	100g banana_80 Black Earl Grey tea_0	Smoked Trout and Cauliflower Rice Salad (p79)_87 30g mixed salad leaves_5 30g cherry tomatoes_7 ¼ tsp olive oil_20 1 tsp sherry vinegar_1	Chickpea Curry (p100)_143 with 1 portion (57g) Kachumber (p223)_10 25g 0% Greek yoghurt, 100g_15 steamed spring greens_20 ¼ tsp nigella seeds_4	unlimited water infused with cucumber slices_0	Dessert Rose (p257)_105
493	50g strawberries_15 25g blueberries_10 50g raspberries_12 60g 0% Greek yoghurt_34	Crayfish and Pear Salad with Dill Dressing (p68)_172	Eggs in Purgatory with Feta, Kale and Capers (p90)_217	Tea made with 15ml semi-skimmed milk_15 unlimited water and herbal tea_0	Miso soup (look for the Yutaka brand which is particularly low calorie)_18
496	Tea made with 30ml semi-skimmed milk_15	Raw Rainbow Salad with Amazingsauce (p220)_97 and Smoked Salmon and Radish Salad (p74)_91	Italian-style Baked Egg (p49)_167 and Cannellini Bean Salad in Little Gem Cups (p81)_93	Tea made with 30ml semi-skimmed milk_15 unlimited fizzy water infused with root ginger and orange slices_0	Miso soup (look for the Yutaka brand which is particularly low calorie)_18

individual calorie count

	Breakfast	Lunch	Dinner	Drinks	Snacks
497	50g 0% Greek yoghurt_29 50g pear_22 50g apple_26 Americano coffee_5 made with 30ml semi-skimmed milk_15	Crab Salad with Toasted Rye Crumbs (p72)_107 Courgette, Chilli and Herb Salad with Feta (p77)_100	King Prawn, Celeriac and Fennel Stew (p154)_159 100g cauliflower rice_34	unlimited water and herbal teas_0	
498	50g 0% Greek yoghurt_29 30g raspberries_7 Black Earl Grey tea_0	Blueberry, Avocado and Corn Salad (p77)_100 with 10g feta_28 2 wholegrain rice cakes with 50g chopped tomato, 30g cottage cheese and basil_86	Vegetable, Butter Bean and Smoked Paprika Stew (p103)_187 with 100g cauliflower rice_34 20g 0% Greek yoghurt_12	unlimited fizzy water infused with fresh mint_0	45g Pico de Gallo (p235)_9 60g celery sticks_6
499	Lebanese-style Breakfast (p38)_145 Black tea_0	Prawn, Mango and Jalapeño Salad (p66)_101 and Courgette, Chilli and Herb Salad with Feta (p77)_100	Chilled Beetroot Soup (p116)_70 50g little gem lettuce_8 with ¼ tsp olive oil_20 5g grated Parmesan cheese_20	Tea made with 30ml semi-skimmed milk_15 unlimited water and herbal tea_0	100g radishes_12 with 1 tsp Za'atar (p228)_8
500	A soft boiled egg with 50g asparagus to dip into it_88	Tomato, Lentil and Broccoli Soup (p106)_178	Lemon Sole with Celeriac Colcannon and Kale (p159)_186 With side salad of 30g mixed salad leaves_5 30g cherry tomatoes_7 ¼ tsp olive oil_20 1 tsp sherry vinegar_1	Tea made with 30ml semi-skimmed milk_15 unlimited water and herbal teas_0	

Calorie Index

Index

〰

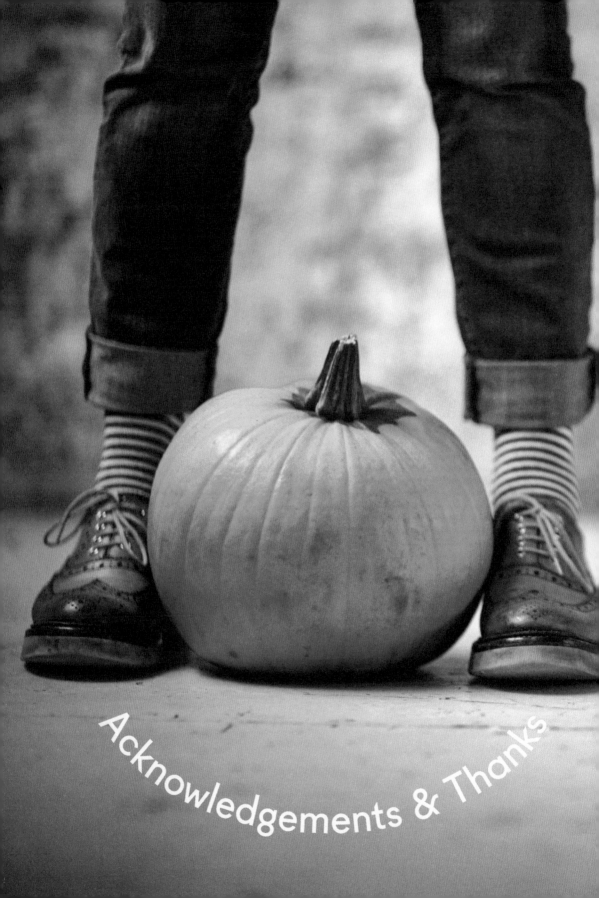

Acknowledgements & Thanks

My first and biggest thanks go to you – to all of you who've supported me and shouted from the rooftops (your keyboards) that you wanted this book. This was a long time coming but everything happens for a reason, my mumma told me, and this book is not the book I would have written three years ago when this all kicked off and I think it was worth the wait. I hope you agree. Thanks for holding on so patiently.

Enormous debt of gratitude to Dr Michael Mosley for kick-starting this whole 5:2 thing and doing the work and research that led to this book happening.

Huge, massive thanks to all my brilliant mates, too. I'm very lucky to be surrounded by strong, clever, creative, brilliant people in my life and I honestly only got through this whole long process with your advice, support and enthusiasm. A book takes a really long time to do – who knew??

Dan – our friendship means the world to me and I honestly don't know what I'd do without you. Thank you for everything and for being by my side every single step of the way.

To my family – this is why I've hardly seen any of you for ages – sorry. Love you all. I'm imagining Grandma Cissie and Grandpa Bob's faces if they could see this book and now I'll never stop crying. I can't believe I forgot to put my roast chicken recipe in, Mumma. Back to texting it to you every other week, I guess.

To my second family – Millie and Joe and the kids – Thank you for letting me stay over and over again while I yo-yo'd my way back and forth between London and Bristol (your home is my favourite place to be).

Cissy – You gave birth to twins as I gave birth to this book and even through the most monumental year of your life, you were there, at the end of the phone, being organised and calm and really bloody smart. Thank you.

To my food babes. To Gizzi – where do I start? You lit the taper and, man, it went off! You're a powerhouse and I owe you so much. Darling Rosie and Ed – so happy and #blessed to have you both as friends.

To my fairy godmother/agent Sheila, and to Becky – You're the best.

To the café babes, and especially Jen. #mindvibes

To Fiona – I only tried the 5:2 because of you and look what happened!! I'm so, so lucky to have you in my life and hope page 202 makes you smile.

To Sam and the Bells crew – massive thanks for all your help and support – the best neighbours I could ever have hoped for while writing my book!

To Ben and to Bev, to Hannah, Charlotte and all at Instyle – you've been big parts of this period – thank you all for everything.

To all those who contributed recipes – Fattie, Jose, Tom – Love you all being in here with me! Thank you! Thanks also to all my Bristol food mates who feature throughout the book – this is the best city in the world and I love being part of our community. You all inspire me.

HUGE thanks and massive respect to the shoot crew – Myles – everyone said 'OH MY GOD YOU'LL LOVE HIM!!' and I did. Marina and Becks – love at first sight. You guys are so, so brilliant and working with you was an absolute joy. Thank you all for all your hard work and being so lovely and making my 'first day at school' wobbles dissipate. Thanks too to Martin, Tab and Lydia, Tom and Fran.

And finally, to the team at HarperCollins – my commissioning editor Carolyn, Orlando, Julie, Sophie and everyone else – I hope I did you proud. Thank you for having faith in me. George and Lucy – your hard work and talent is so apparent in this book and I'm immensely grateful to both of you. We did a book, guys!!!!

Now, let's eat.

Thorsons
An imprint of HarperCollins*Publishers*
1 London Bridge Street
London SE1 9GF

www.harpercollins.co.uk

First published by Thorsons 2016

1 2 3 4 5 6 7 8 9 10

Text © Elly Curshen 2016
Photography © Myles New 2016

Elly Curshen asserts the moral right to
be identified as the author of this work

A catalogue record of this book is
available from the British Library

Food styling: Marina Filippelli
Props styling: Lydia Brun &
Tabitha Hawkins
Nutritional Analysis: Elsa Robson

ISBN: 978-0-00-815792-0

Printed and bound in Spain by
Gráficas Estella, S.L.

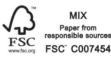

MIX
Paper from
responsible sources
FSC
www.fsc.org   FSC™ C007454

FSC™ is a non-profit international organisation established to promote the
responsible management of the world's forests. Products carrying the FSC
label are independently certified to assure consumers that they come from
forests that are managed to meet the social, economic and ecological needs
of present and future generations, and other controlled sources.

Find out more about HarperCollins and the environment at
www.harpercollins.co.uk/green